"Tim's book is filled with great advic
It's well worth following and applyin
way we are supposed to."

Dr. Caroline Leaf, cognitive neuroscientist,
communication pathologist, and author

"Guided by his strong faith and extensive scientific knowledge, Dr. Jennings has provided a well-researched and commonsense book aimed at helping one understand the complexities of dementia, while offering recommendations for maintaining healthy brain function into our later years."

Rodney A. Poling, MD, DFAPA, medical director, Behavioral Healthcare
Center, Columbia, Tennessee; board-certified geriatric psychiatrist

"Your brain may age, but it does not have to get old. Dr. Jennings clearly describes how to practically manage the medical and lifestyle variables that can positively impact brain health and the process of aging. Age is a number, but getting old is a lifestyle."

Michael Lyles, psychiatrist, author, and speaker

"Memory concerns and age-related cognitive losses are some of the most significant issues we face as we age. Those who desire improved brain and general health should read Dr. Timothy Jennings's book *The Aging Brain*. In addition to providing a comprehensive review of normal brain aging, Dr. Jennings translates data from recent scientific studies into practical strategies for improving memory and other cognitive skills. By following the suggested lifestyle changes one may prevent the occurrence of Alzheimer's disease."

Allan A. Anderson, MD, medical director, Bratton
Memory Clinic, Easton, Maryland; assistant professor,
Johns Hopkins School of Medicine; former president,
The American Association for Geriatric Psychiatry

"I read everything Dr. Jennings writes; he is on the leading edge of what we need to know for long-term brain vibrancy and health. Read these pages; you will be personally helped. I was."

Dr. Gregg Jantz

"Brain-health research is exploding, and it's important to each and every one of us. From childhood development to late-life challenges such as dementia, brain function is at the center of everything. Few life issues are as painful as watching someone you love deteriorate mentally. Dr. Jennings helps us understand the aging brain, offering timely wisdom, practical insight, guidance, and wise counsel. This book is a wonderful addition to your personal and professional library and ministry resources."

Dr. Tim Clinton, president, American Association of Christian Counselors

"If you are like me, with a family history of dementia or Alzheimer's, then you are intrigued by this book because it addresses an area of fear in your life. Experiencing the ravages of these diseases up close and personal, we likely share a fear that our brain will somehow let us down before our body does. Having also been to some of Dr. Jennings's workshops and having my own fascination with the brain, I was more than eager to read his manuscript. And now that I have soaked up every single word, I can attest to this being one of the most valuable books I've ever read. It will most certainly be a recommended read to my clients, who will benefit from the scientific explanations and practical applications provided. I trust you will also find hope in these pages."

Donna Gibbs, author of *Becoming Resilient* and the upcoming publication, *Silencing Insecurities*; director, A Clear Word Counseling Center

"Someone once said, 'The hero you should be chasing is who you will be ten years from now.' We all wonder what we will be like in ten or twenty years. As we age we wonder if we will live long, healthy lives. Tim Jennings addresses our concerns and fears about the aging process and details precise guidelines to ensure a better and healthier future you. As one who has faced the challenge of Alzheimer's disease with an aging parent, I found this book to be a hopeful and encouraging lesson in breaking that genetic chain. This book will inspire you to become your future hero."

Aaron Fruh, author of *Bounce: Learning to Thrive through Loss, Tragedy, and Heartache*

THE
AGING
BRAIN

THE
AGING
BRAIN

PROVEN STEPS TO PREVENT DEMENTIA
AND SHARPEN YOUR MIND

TIMOTHY R. JENNINGS, MD

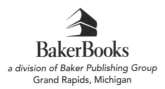

BakerBooks

a division of Baker Publishing Group
Grand Rapids, Michigan

Published by Baker Books
a division of Baker Publishing Group
PO Box 6287, Grand Rapids, MI 49516-6287
www.bakerbooks.com

Printed in the United States of America

Library of Congress Cataloging-in-Publication Data
Names: Jennings, Timothy R., 1961– author.
Title: The aging brain : proven steps to prevent dementia and sharpen your mind / Timothy R. Jennings MD.
Description: Grand Rapids : Baker Publishing Group, 2018. | Includes bibliographical references.
Identifiers: LCCN 2017060002 | ISBN 9780801075223 (pbk.)
Subjects: LCSH: Dementia—Prevention. | Lifestyles.
Classification: LCC RC521 .J46 2018 | DDC 616.8/31—dc23
LC record available at https://lccn.loc.gov/2017060002

18   19   20   21   22   23   24   7   6   5   4   3

CONTENTS

7

AUTHOR'S NOTE

This book proposes specific lifestyle interventions to improve health, slow aging, and reduce the risk of late-onset Alzheimer's disease (AD). This book is not intended to provide steps to address other types of dementia, such as frontotemporal dementia, Lewy body dementia, spongiform disorders, and so on. You should consult a qualified medical professional before initiating these interventions or any other fitness regimen. The interventions in this book are intended to be implemented in consultation with your doctor, and this is especially so if you suffer from any medical condition.

ACKNOWLEDGMENTS

I want to thank my wife, Christie, who always supports me during the many hours I spend in research and writing. Christie—I couldn't do it without you!

I also want to express my thanks to my editor, Jamie Chavez, who had the difficult task of slogging through the rough draft and helping me break down a lot of scientific facts into bite-size, understandable, and actionable bits. Jamie—thanks for your help. I needed it.

INTRODUCTION

It's Personal

This book is personal—not simply because my heart has been touched by the numerous patients I have treated over the last twenty-six years, many of whom suffered from dementia, nor because my wife and I are in our middle fifties and acutely aware of the difficulties of aging but because over the last several years I have watched my wife's mother slowly being ravaged by Alzheimer's disease. I have felt the heartache, the frustration, and the sadness as she has become more feeble, less aware, and less capable. I know the utter frustration of being helpless as a loved one, who had been so reliable, so strong, and such a bastion of courage and support to everyone else, slowly loses the ability to care for her most basic needs.

I have seen the hurt on my wife's face as she recognized each newly lost ability and found her mother becoming ever less present, and my heart is torn every time I see the fear in my wife's eyes as she realizes her risk of dementia is increased because her mother has it.

Yes, this book is personal. In writing it I have sought not only good scientific evidence but also usable information to be put into practical action that will promote better health and slow aging and help us in the pursuit of our goal to prevent the development of late-onset Alzheimer's disease—even in those who are at higher risk for developing it and in those who are already showing early signs of impairment!

It's been said that beautiful young people are accidents of nature, but beautiful old people are works of art. I dedicate this book to my wife, Christie, who is both a beautiful "accident of nature" and the most beautiful work of art I have ever known. Christie, I hope this book will remove your fear and give you confidence to know that rather than slowly fading away you can grow more beautiful every day!

And to the reader, I invite you to share in this vision, to use the information in this book to not only live long but also live well and grow more beautiful every day!

PART 1

HISTORY AND AGING

1

The Problem of Aging

We All Do It

And yet the wiser mind
Mourns less for what age takes away
Than what it leaves behind.

William Wordsworth, "The Fountain, a
Conversation," in *Lyrical Ballads*, 1800

It was painful to watch, agonizing really. Anger, frustration, help-lessness, mixed with sadness, heartache, loss—and of course denial, this can't be happening. But sadly it was.

The features were the same—blue eyes, teeth yellowed from years of use—but her historically warm and friendly smile wasn't warm, wasn't friendly, not anymore. Like so much of her, it was empty, just a shell—she was a wasting, shriveling, slowly decaying shell.

"Hello, Mom," was met with a confused look. Her formerly thick brunette hair, always kept, was now thinning, snow white, and disheveled. How could this be happening? Alzheimer's disease—the name given to this destroyer of worlds, the thief that neuron by neuron slowly steals life away. Like a picture slowly fading, like the last beams of sunlight growing ever dimmer, this insidious disease robs a person not only of ability but also of their very selves.

In the twenty-first century Alzheimer's disease is perhaps the most frightening diagnosis a person can receive. But it has not always been this way. In fact, dementias like Alzheimer's are a relatively new problem for humanity. Just fifty years ago cancer was the most dreaded diagnosis for many. While cancer remains a terrible problem, for those over fifty the threat of losing oneself as the brain slowly deteriorates is even more terrifying. The rise of dementias as a problem in human history is a result of ever improving health care and the fact that people are living longer. Prior to the last one hundred years few lived long enough to develop dementia.

Throughout history there have always been health scares, but dementia wasn't one of them. During the fourteenth century the Black Death (bubonic plague) swept across Europe, killing one-third of the population. People lived in terror of contracting this mysterious disease. No one understood the cause, let alone how to treat it. Religious leaders proclaimed the ghastly destruction was the wrath of an offended god. Yet it was merely a bacterial infection (*Yersinia pestis*) carried by fleas. Today the disease occurs infrequently, and if antibiotics are given, it rarely results in death.

The greatest killers throughout most of human history have been infections—from either disease or wounds. Prior to modern antibiotics and sanitation, life expectancy was short. Before the twentieth century, essentially every family lost children in death. Before 1900 only 39 percent of men and 43 percent of women lived to be sixty-five years of age, but by 1997, 77 percent of men and 86 percent of women lived to the age of sixty-five.[1]

At the turn of the twentieth century (1900), the top three causes of death, accounting for 30 percent of all deaths, were from infections: pneumonia and influenza, tuberculosis, and gastro-intestinal infections (diarrhea and enteritis). But by 1990, with the advent of water treatment, food inspections, antibiotics, modern dentistry, and childhood vaccinations, this had markedly changed. No longer were large segments of the populace dying from infections. By 1990 the top three killers, accounting for 60 percent of all deaths, were heart disease, cancer, and stroke.[2]

Today's top killers are as follows:

- Cardiovascular disease—28.2 percent
- Cancer—22.2 percent
- Stroke—6.6 percent
- Chronic lung disease—6.2 percent
- Alzheimer's disease—4.2 percent
- Diabetes—2.9 percent
- Flu and pneumonia—2.6 percent
- Accidental injury—2.2 percent

Strikingly, the top five causes of death are all a result of people living longer—they are no longer dying at a young age from infections. America as a populous is aging, and with an aging population comes increased numbers of age-related diseases. In 1950 there were twelve million people over the age of sixty-five accounting for 8 percent of the population. By 2002 this increased to 12 percent or thirty-six million people. And according to the Centers for Disease Control and Prevention (CDC), by 2030 there will be seventy-one million people in the United States over the age of sixty-five.

The number of very old, those over eighty-five, is also increasing. From 1950 to 2002 there has been an eightfold increase in the number of people ages eighty-five and older. It is projected that by 2020 there will be seven million people over the age of eighty-five, and by 2040 that number will double to fourteen million.[3]

For the young the idea of living longer is all about length of years, but as we grow older the quality of life begins to overshadow mere age. This is evidenced by the growing right-to-die trend—the principle that individuals have the right to end their lives, usually because their quality of life has become so poor it is tantamount to sustained torture. In the United States, three state legislatures (Oregon, Washington, and Vermont) have passed laws permitting physician-assisted suicide, and in 2009 Montana's Supreme Court ruled physician-assisted suicide legal. In California in 2015 the governor signed a physician-assisted suicide law into effect during a special session of the legislature after the law failed to pass in regular session. Its full implementation is pending at the time of the writing of this book.

Pain, suffering, and disability undermine quality of life and must be considered in any discussion of aging. In 2011 there were more than 40 million people ages sixty-five and older in the United States, and more than 14.5 million (36.6 percent) of them suffered with some type of disability. More than 9 million (23.6 percent) had impairments in their ability to walk, nearly 6.5 million (16.2 percent) could not live independently, more than 6 million (15 percent) had impaired hearing, nearly 3.8 million (9.4 percent) were disabled due to cognitive impairment, more than 3.5 million (8.9 percent) could no longer provide basic self-care, and more than 2.6 million (6.8 percent) were visually disabled.[4]

People don't simply want to live longer; they want to live better—healthier, happier, and fuller lives. The greater question today is not how do we live longer but how do we live better—how do we retain our vitality, health, independence, and autonomy? How do we slow the ravages of time?

The good news is not only can we live longer but we can also live better, healthier, and more vibrant lives. By making the right choices we can maintain our independence, vitality, and most importantly our mental acuity. Dementias such as Alzheimer's disease are not inevitable. Disability is not predestined. Yes, we can live longer, and we can live better!

In this book we will explore aging. I'll differentiate normal aging from pathological aging. I will identify activities that accelerate aging and increase the risk of both physical disability and dementia, but I'll also provide specific actions a person can take to slow the aging process and protect our brains and bodies from deterioration in order to maintain our independence, autonomy, and abilities as we age. At the end of each chapter will be lists of learning points or action steps or both for you to implement that are designed to reduce your risk of dementia. Because of individual differences from person to person, not every intervention is applicable to every person. For instance, a person with nut allergies would not benefit from adding nuts to their diet whereas those without the allergy would. Select those elements from the action steps that are applicable to your life and build an action plan that will improve your vitality and brain health and keep your mind sharp.

Science and medicine have reduced the risk of dying young; now it is up to us to decide how we will age. Will we make purposeful choices to maximize health and maintain our abilities?

My wish for you is that you will use the information in this book not only to live longer but also to live more vibrantly with each passing year!

▪ LEARNING POINTS ▪

1. Modern science has reduced the risk of dying young.
2. Dementia is a problem of living longer.
3. We can make choices to reduce the risk of dementia even while living longer.

2

Developing a Healthy Brain

It Needs a Healthy Body

A comfortable old age is the reward of a well-spent youth. Instead of its bringing sad and melancholy prospects of decay, it should give us hopes of eternal youth in a better world.

Ray Palmer (1808–87), American
clergyman and poet

When we talk about aging, what do we mean? Are we speaking merely of chronologically growing older or do we mean something else? While a common dictionary definition of *aging* is the length of time something or someone lives or exists, in this book when we speak of aging we are not referring merely to the number of years one lives but also to the slow decline in vitality, health, and ability that occurs as we age. Most people would be thrilled to live eternally if they knew they would retain their health, vitality, strength, and abilities. Aging in the context of this book refers to *functional aging*—the slow decline in vitality and ability.

While time passes at a constant rate for every person, not every person ages at the same rate. Life experiences and the choices we make affect our passage through time and can slow or accelerate our aging—the gradual loss of vitality and ability.

In this book we will identify multiple factors that accelerate aging—and interventions we can take to slow it down. While we will discover there are many factors involved, this does not need to be overwhelming. Consider for a moment those factors that contribute to your car either breaking down or being disabled by an accident. These factors are analogous to what can happen in our bodies.

- Poor construction (e.g., ignition switch problems that contribute to accidents[1])—genetic or epigenetic vulnerabilities to aging
- Poor condition—lack of exercise or failure to maintain healthy nutrition
- Defective or worn-out brakes—impaired ability to calm down or slow down
- Bald tires—overly emotional individuals who are not grounded in reality or who easily slip and slide as the emotional weather changes
- Distractions (e.g., texting, changing the radio station, other people in the vehicle)—caught up in entertainment or alcohol and drug addictions such that one doesn't attend to one's health
- Poor visibility—lack of education, insight, or understanding
- Wet, snowy, or icy conditions—toxins, pollution, and industrial exposures that accelerate aging
- Purposeful sabotage—physical and emotional abuse, war, and crime

- Sleeping at the wheel—failure to listen and learn; ignoring healthy guidance when presented

Just as each factor above contributes to the risk of your car breaking down or being wrecked, so too each of the corresponding bodily factors contributes to our risk of disability as we age. Addressing one or more of the factors related to our cars does not guarantee we will avoid a breakdown or accident, nor does having one or more of these problems make accidents or breakdowns a certainty. However, the more of these problems that exist simultaneously, the greater is the likelihood that an accident or breakdown will occur. Every factor that we address reduces risk. Likewise, when it comes to aging we will explore many factors that accelerate aging. The more of these factors we address, the more vitality we retain and the greater we are able to slow the aging process and reduce our risk of dementia.

A Healthy Brain Requires a Healthy Body

The first principle to maintaining a youthful brain is to maintain a healthy body. Why is it important to maintain physical health if one wants a healthy brain? Because the primary purpose of every organ system of the body is to serve the brain: the lungs breathe and the heart beats in order to provide oxygen and nutrients to the brain. The legs move the brain from place to place while the arms allow the brain to interact with the world. The primary function of our eyes and ears is to provide data input to the brain.

The gastrointestinal (GI) system absorbs nutrients to provide energy and raw materials for the operation of the entire body but especially for the brain. While the brain weighs only three pounds, which is about 1–2 percent of the body weight, it utilizes 20 percent of the body's energy. The GI system also protects the brain from potential toxins. Whatever we eat and drink is absorbed into the *blood.* But before the blood carries what has been ingested to the brain it first passes through the liver. This is so the liver can identify and neutralize any toxins and poisons to prevent them from impairing or damaging the brain. For instance, the liver has enzymes that detoxify alcohol. In order to get intoxicated, a person has to drink enough alcohol to overwhelm the liver's ability to detoxify it. Ingesting small amounts of alcohol will not affect the brain because the liver will detoxify it so that it will never reach the brain.

When we understand this reality we realize that whatever undermines the health of the body will necessarily undermine the health and functioning of the brain. Not surprisingly, studies have shown that major illnesses such as anemia,[2] diabetes mellitus,[3] and cardiovascular disease[4] all increase the risk of developing dementia later in life. What is less commonly known is that failing to care for one's teeth increases the risk of developing dementia.[5] In fact, research has found that those "with the fewest teeth had the highest risk of prevalence and incidence of dementia."[6] So a simple action to reduce dementia risk is to practice good oral hygiene—daily brushing, flossing, and regular dental checkups—all focused on keeping your teeth and gums healthy. It is impossible to keep our brains healthy without keeping our bodies healthy.

Design Law

One idea we must understand and that is crucial for being able to make healthy life choices is the idea of living in harmony with design law. What is design law? Simply stated, design laws are those parameters, protocols, and principles on which life is constructed to operate. In this context they are commonly known as the laws of health. Why don't we put water in the gas tanks of our cars? It is so much cheaper than gasoline; think of all the money we could save. Will the manufacturer inflict punishment if we fail to follow the written instructions in the owner's manual? Why don't we do it? The reason is quite simple—the vehicle was not *designed* to run on water and therefore will break down.

Design laws are those laws that govern the operation of the fabric of reality itself, such as the law of gravity, the laws of thermodynamics, physics, and health. Human beings cannot create space, time, matter, energy, or life. But thinking in this way is counter to how most human organizations function. Human beings make up rules in an attempt to bring order, which we call laws, and then enforce those rules with threats of punishment.

Thinking that is counter to design laws is so automatic that many people fail to realize it just doesn't work when it comes to healthful living. Adolescents often think that what makes tobacco or marijuana smoking wrong is that it is illegal; if the laws change then smoking these toxins will be okay. They fail to understand the difference between human laws and design laws. Humans can pass laws to make cigarettes and marijuana legal, but we can never pass laws to make them healthy! Regardless of whether smoking is legal, tobacco smokers are violating the laws of health and cannot escape the damaging results.

Many patients live like adolescents, thinking very little of design laws, eating and drinking anything they want, and then expecting the doctor to provide a pill to resolve the damage. Life and health simply do not work this way.

We will come back to the idea of design law many times in this book. But for now, simply understand this: *It is not possible to be healthy outside the laws of health.* Understanding design law, especially how it applies to our physical and mental health, is critical to slowing the aging process and maximizing our vitality and wellness.

Take a moment to review your own life and lifestyle and answer this question: Am I currently engaging in any practice or activity that I *know* is unhealthy for me? If the answer is yes, consider why—what is the reason you are doing it? And consider the price you are paying, not just the monetary price but more importantly the price to your health, wellness, and vitality. If you want to slow the aging process, examine your life and choose to eliminate practices that you already know are unhealthy. I am speaking here of ongoing practices—the routine, habitual, repetitive engagement in activities that are unhealthy—not the occasional indulgence. Having a Thanksgiving feast once a year will not have a significant negative health effect if throughout the rest of the year one eats reasonably. However, a healthy meal once a year or once a month won't provide any significant health benefits if the daily routine is a junk-food diet.

The Brain

The brain is an amazing organ composed of over one hundred billion neurons and over one trillion supporting cells. Each neuron can have up to ten thousand connections to other neurons, and it is these interconnections that are critical to intelligence and information processing.

But what determines whether a person has a complex interconnected brain capable of critical reasoning, problem solving, and real wisdom, or a brain that prunes, deletes, or simply fails to develop its circuitry? The most critical time for brain growth is during fetal development and early childhood. During fetal development the brain is in production mode, cranking out the raw materials and weaving them together to form the various foundational structures and networks of the brain. At certain points in development tens of thousands of brains cells are being produced per second, and then, after production, all these billions of cells have to assemble and organize in their appropriate locations in order to form the networks needed for normal functioning. Therefore, fetal development is a very vulnerable time period for brain development.

Recently, news reports have documented the devastating impact the Zika virus has on fetal brain development. What appears to be happening is that the Zika virus hijacks the brain's factory cells (the cells that produce the billions of other cells), and instead of producing brain cells these factory cells crank out more Zika virus. Thus, fetuses infected with Zika are born with severely small brains and heads. But many other factors can also negatively impact normal fetal brain development—alcohol, tobacco, environmental toxins, malnutrition of the mother, and infections. So the first factor in determining whether a person develops a brain with complex interconnections is a healthy experience in the womb. While it is obviously too late for those of us reading this book to change our prebirth experiences, it is not too late to share this information with our children and grandchildren and thereby provide benefit to future generations.

Regardless of what happened before birth, once a person is born into the world the brain remains pliable and changeable. In fact, the first seven to eight years of childhood are critical in establishing networks that form a foundation for future learning and behavior. When a child is born into the world the brain has millions more neurons than that brain will have by age eight. The first eight years of life are a time of rapid brain wiring, reshaping, and developing. Ideas, abilities, concepts, and beliefs are being wired into the brain. What determines which circuits develop and which do not? Whether those neural circuits are utilized or not, which is a function of another design law—the law of exertion.

The law of exertion is simply this: if you want something to get stronger you *must* exercise it. If you want strong muscles you must exercise them, if you want strong musical ability you must practice your instrument, if you want strong math skills you must work problems. When exercised, the brain fires neurons that correspond to the specific activity. The repeated firing of these neurons results in not only the retention of the corresponding neurons but also the production of new neurons and the recruitment of other neurons—and the circuitry for that ability expands. The brain structure changes based on the choices we make in thinking, acting, and experiencing. But if you don't use it, you lose it.

Persons born blind have been shown to have heightened ability to process other sensory information, greater memory, and greater cognitive processing. Recent brain mapping comparing the brains of individuals born blind with those of persons who were blinded later in life found that the brains of those born without sight had recruited areas of the visual cortex to help process the sensory input of touch, smell, and hearing.[7] The brain is not a static organ; it is highly pliable and in a constant state of flux based on life experience.

While the brain continues to rewire and change throughout life, these changes are made more easily during the first eight years of life. Imagine a blank whiteboard versus one filled with drawings. It is easier to establish a new drawing on a blank board than on one already filled with drawings. To create new images on a board filled with drawings one has to erase the previous drawings. Likewise, it is easier to learn in childhood when the brain is "blank." Once patterns of learning are established, new learning can and does take place, but one often has to "unlearn" in order to learn new things. Many golfers understand it is easier to learn to correctly swing the club right from the beginning than to try to learn the correct swing after already having established a "bad" swing.

This is a book about aging; why then are we talking about early childhood? Because it is in early childhood that the foundations for our future lives are set. One of the factors that has been demonstrated to slow brain aging and the risk of dementia is education and mental activity—that is, learning new things. This is a direct function of the law of exertion. Education exercises the brain and results in its development. Those who are educated develop more complex brains and are generally more knowledgeable about how to live healthy lives, thus avoiding many destructive factors that accelerate aging. As a result they are more resilient and resistant to the ravages of time. And studies have confirmed this. Those with sixteen years or more of education can expect to live more than a decade longer than those who did not graduate from high school.[8]

In order to stimulate brain pliability—the branching and connecting of new circuits and the formation of new neurons—the brain has a group of proteins that stimulate neuronal production, sprouting, and growth. These are called *neurotrophic factors*. Think of them as fertilizer for the brain. When these proteins are available the brain circuits remain healthy and flexible, and new learning is easier. But when these factors are not available learning becomes more difficult, and the brain will actually wither and shrink.

Three known neurotrophins are brain-derived neurotrophic factor (BDNF), vascular endothelial growth factor (VEGF), and nerve growth factor (NGF). These brain fertilizers are *shut down* by factors that accelerate aging such as fear and worry, tobacco, illegal drugs, heavy alcohol use, sedentary lifestyle, mood disorders, unhealthy diet, oxidative stress, and chronic pain. While certain medications have been shown to affect individual neurotrophic factors, only physical exercise turns on all three—the law of exertion! And the benefits of exercise to brain pliability are not restricted to our childhood. In fact, persons over age sixty-five who exercise (walk) as little as fifteen minutes per day have been shown to experience 2 percent growth in the brain's primary memory cortex (hippocampus), which effectively reversed two years of aging.[9]

Childhood with its rapid brain changes is a period when the brain is extremely pliable and changeable. The activities, education, nutrition, and religious practices experienced in childhood will impact the structural development of the brain. Adverse events will negatively affect brain development because they increase activity in stress pathways, which cause alterations in gene expression and result in individuals with increased risk of physical and mental health problems later in life, thereby accelerating aging and increasing the risk of an early death.[10]

We cannot go back and undo our childhoods but because the brain remains changeable throughout our entire lives, we can make decisions today that will protect our brains, slow the aging process, and reduce our risk of dementia.

The body and brain are intimately connected, and brain health cannot be maintained without maintaining the health of the body. The brain is truly an amazing organ, and throughout this book we will document how you can keep your brain in peak working condition!

▪ LEARNING POINTS ▪

1. Aging is the slow loss of vitality and ability.
2. Life operates on design laws—laws of health. Understanding and living in harmony with these design parameters is essential for maintaining healthy functioning. Deviation from these parameters is damaging and accelerates aging and loss of vitality and ability.
3. One of the design laws is the law of exertion—if you want something to get stronger you must exercise it. If you don't use it, you will lose it.
4. Every organ system of the body has as its primary purpose to serve the brain. Thus, healthy brain function requires maintaining as optimal physical health as possible.
5. The human brain is in a constant state of flux, changing itself based on the choices we make and the experiences we encounter. We therefore have the ability to choose experiences and actions that will slow the aging process and promote healthy brain development and function.

▪ ACTION PLAN: THINGS TO DO ▪

1. Practice good oral hygiene: brush, floss, and get regular dental checkups.

2. Establish a relationship with a primary care physician and get annual physical exams; work with your doctor to prevent and/or treat any physical health problems.

3. Inventory your life and identify practices you *know* are unhealthy, and then make changes that move you toward healthier lifestyle practices. (We will examine many specific examples in later chapters.)

4. Share with family and friends who are planning on having children the importance of a healthy pregnancy and early childhood to the development of a healthy brain.

5. Engage in lifelong learning, contemplate new ideas, challenge yourself to see issues from a different vantage point, join discussion groups, take art lessons, join a Bible study—the list of possibilities is endless. Engage your mind regularly!

6. Begin walking twenty minutes each day. (We will explore physical exercise in more detail in a later chapter.)

3

Epigenetics and Aging

The Impact from Our Ancestors

People will not look forward to posterity, who
never look backward to their ancestors.

Edmund Burke, *Reflections on the
Revolution in France,* 1790

While most of this book will explore various factors
that impact aging over which we have significant influence, the complete story of aging begins before we
are even conceived. In this chapter we will explore those influences
originating in our immediate ancestors that affect gene expression
and impact aging in us. While we can do nothing to change history and the genetic material with which we were born, we can
through healthy choices not only alter our genetic expression and
thus impact our own health but also pass those changes down to
our children, grandchildren, and great-grandchildren, impacting
their health as well.

Every cell of our body that contains a nucleus contains the same genetic information—deoxyribonucleic acid, or DNA (with the exception of individuals with extremely rare disorders). Yet bone cells are different from skin cells, which are different from muscle cells, which are different from the cells in our eyes that transform light into electrical energy so we can see or the cells on our tongues that transform chemical signals into electrical ones so we can taste. Yes, all the cells in a person's body have the same DNA, but the DNA is *expressed* differently, resulting in wide diversity in the shape, structure, and function of the various types of tissues throughout the body.

Our DNA is like a vast library of information with instructions on how to build everything the body needs. But each cell type opens only the books (genes) in the library that contain the information those cells need to do their job. Thus, cells in the stomach do not access the information on how to make bone, and cells in the brain don't access the information on how to make blood cells, and so on. All the information is there in the library (chromosomes in the nucleus of each cell), but cells open only the books (genes) that have the information they need. This means there must be some instructions directing the cells on which books (genes) to access and use.

It was in 1957 that researcher Conrad Wadddington first made this observation and hypothesized that there must be some set of instructions that sits above the DNA instructing the DNA on which genes to turn on (express) and which genes to turn off (not express). He coined the term *epigenetics—epi* means above as in *epi*dermis (the top layer of your skin), and genetics refers to the DNA. So *epigenetics* means the chemical instructions that direct the access and usage of the information contained within the DNA.

DNA, though incredibly small, is the massively huge database of information in which the instructions on how to build every part of our bodies are stored. Imagine a zipper, two rows of teeth that interlock. Now imagine that zipper is very long—miles long.

It is zipped, then sections are wrapped around spools, and those spools are packed tightly together. This would be similar to how our DNA is stored. Each tooth on the zipper represents a DNA molecule. The molecules are organized in a way to create coded information from which our bodies are built. (Imagine the DNA molecules are letters of the alphabet, and they are organized to spell words that are put together in sentences containing building instructions for the body.) Just as there are two sides to a zipper, there are two strands of DNA that zip together, then wrap around histone molecules, which are packed tightly together to form our chromosomes. But in order to read the code the zipper must unpack, unwind, and unzip. DNA expression is modified by either enhancing or impairing the unpacking, unwinding, and unzipping.

There are various molecules that can attach to the DNA and influence its expression at these various points. For instance, methyl groups can attach directly to the DNA strand, and when this happens the DNA in that region is locked down. This would be like getting a shirttail caught in your zipper—the zipper cannot unzip. Methyl groups, therefore, when attached to the DNA strand, shut down the expression of the DNA in the region where they attach. Conversely, any gene that had methyl groups removed would experience an increase in expression. Environmental factors, life experiences, and even the thoughts we think can impact how our DNA is being expressed. And when we have children we not only pass along our DNA sequences but also the epigenetic instructions specifying which genes are turned on and which genes are shut down.

Smoking, Famine, and Grandchildren

Researchers in Sweden discovered that men who began smoking before age eleven had altered genes carried on their Y chromosome that caused their grandsons to have greater likelihood of obesity than if they had not smoked. And individuals who in their childhood (before puberty) experienced a short food supply had altered DNA expression such that the men conferred greater mortality risk to their grandsons and the women conferred greater mortality risk to their granddaughters. This means if you are a man and your grandfather (or if a woman and your grandmother) experienced a significant famine in their childhood, then you began life with a greater risk of dying young than if your grandparent had a normal food supply.[1]

Low-Calorie Diet during Pregnancy

Another provocative study examined children born in the Netherlands during WWII when there was a severe food shortage and whose mothers averaged about five hundred calories of food intake per day. These children grew up to have higher rates of obesity, diabetes mellitus type 2, and other metabolic problems such as hypercholesterolemia than their siblings (of the same parents) who were born when normal amounts of food were available. Genetic examination found that the metabolically compromised individuals had 5 percent fewer methyl caps on one specific gene (*IGF2*). This would result in an increased expression of this specific gene. The researchers concluded that this gene is involved in food metabolism, and the increased expression resulted in these individuals extracting more energy from food than their siblings.

What appears to have happened is that when these individuals were in utero during the food shortage, a signal was sent to the developing fetus that there were not many nutritional resources in the world. This low-energy input resulted in fewer methyl caps attached to gene *IGF2*, and these individuals were born genetically programmed to get more energy out of food. But the war ended and food supply normalized, and with normal food intake these individuals experienced greater rates of obesity, diabetes, and other metabolic problems—all of which, as we will see in later chapters, accelerate aging and increase the risk of dementia and early demise.[2] Though we cannot alter the conditions of our birth, we can choose to alter our dietary patterns to conform to our individual ability to extract energy from food and thereby avoid or resolve obesity, diabetes, and hypercholesterolemia, slow our aging, and reduce our risk of dementia.

Smoking, Pregnancy, and Epigenetics

People have known for several decades that smoking during pregnancy is damaging to the developing fetus and increases the risk of smaller babies, learning and behavior problems, sudden infant death syndrome, and mental illness.[3] But in 2016 researchers discovered that smoking while pregnant has much more devastating effects on the genetic expression of the child than imagined. Smoking while pregnant epigenetically alters more than six thousand genes, and nearly three thousand of these alterations persist into later life. Some of these altered genes have been implicated in cleft palate, asthma, and contributing to various cancers, including lung, colorectal, and liver.[4] At least one study found that girls who were exposed to tobacco smoke in the womb were two to three times more likely to become nicotine addicted if exposed to tobacco later in life than girls not exposed to tobacco smoke in utero.[5] This means that mothers who smoked while pregnant altered the reward pathways in the brains of their daughters, making them more vulnerable to nicotine addiction later in life. And as I will document later in this book, tobacco use accelerates aging and contributes to increased risk of dementia.

Alcohol, Pregnancy, and Epigenetics

Likewise we have known for generations that heavy alcohol consumption while pregnant increases the risk of all types of health problems—from fetal alcohol syndrome with multiple organ defects to increasing risks of mental illness.[6] Many of these problems are a result of epigenetic modification and accelerate aging later in life. But what if a woman drank only one alcoholic beverage per week while pregnant? Would such a small quantity of alcohol have an impact on her unborn child? The answer appears to be yes. Children born to women who drank one alcoholic beverage per week had smaller heads, were shorter, and had more behavior and emotional problems later in life than those whose mothers did not drink.[7] Again, these effects occur through epigenetic changes, and as we will see in later chapters, unresolved emotional stress accelerates the aging process.

If you find the taste of alcohol particularly enjoyable, perhaps your mother drank while pregnant with you. Animal research has documented that if a mother drank alcohol while pregnant, epigenetic modifications occurred in the genes of her offspring that code for taste, and her children would experience that alcohol tastes better than if she had not drank while pregnant.[8] As we will discover in later chapters, heavy alcohol use accelerates aging and increases risk of dementia.

Air Pollution, Pregnancy, and Epigenetics

Dr. Bradley Peterson and his fellow researchers discovered that exposure to air pollution while pregnant impacts brain development. They found a dose-dependent effect of the concentration of air pollution on the developing fetal brain that altered white-matter tracks in the left hemisphere, resulting in increased risk of attention deficit hyperactivity disorder (ADHD) in the offspring. This means the greater the exposure to polycyclic aromatic hydrocarbons (the pollution from burning fossil fuels), the greater the damage to the white-matter tracks and the more likely a person will experience ADHD later in life.[9] ADHD impacts the ability to organize, plan, self-restrain, and complete tasks. Those with untreated ADHD have higher rates of substance use problems, more relationship conflicts, and experience greater stress from routine life activities—all of which accelerate aging and increase the risk of dementia.

Mother's Thinking While Pregnant and the Fetal Brain

Not only do diet, alcohol, tobacco, and pollution impact our genetic expression, but also the mother's thinking patterns and stress levels epigenetically alter gene expression in the developing fetal brain, increasing the risk of depression and anxiety later in life.

One study of more than four thousand mothers and their children who were followed for eighteen years found that if the mother had a pattern of pessimistic, negative, and depressive thinking while pregnant it increased the risk of her child developing depression eighteen years later by 21 percent.[10] This association remained after accounting for other maternal and offspring risk factors for depression. And those with a history of depression have a higher risk of developing dementia than those who have not had depression.

Another study found that if a mother is highly stressed while pregnant, which may be no fault of her own, then her child will be born with a brain more vulnerable to anxiety and depression. A nineteen-year-old woman whose husband gets deployed into combat will be stressed. A twenty-five-year-old woman whose mother gets diagnosed with late-stage cancer will be stressed. The increased stress may not be due to unhealthy thinking patterns in the mother. But for whatever reason, if a woman is highly stressed during pregnancy, her stress hormones (glucocorticoids) will cross the placental barrier, cross the developing fetal blood-brain barrier, and epigenetically alter the braking mechanism in the developing fetal-stress circuitry (amygdala). This results in a child born with a more sensitive anxiety circuitry and an impaired braking mechanism to calm the anxiety circuitry. Such children are born more anxiety prone and less capable of calming themselves than if their mothers had not been highly stressed during pregnancy.[11] As we will explore in later chapters, unremitting anxiety, stress, and depression increase inflammatory cascades, which accelerate aging and increase the risk of depression and dementia.

Early Childhood and Epigenetics

What we have learned thus far is that before we are born factors impact our DNA and contribute to the aging process. Such factors work together to establish our starting point, our biological and genetic state at birth. However, our genes and thus our bodies and brains remain changeable based on experiences throughout our lives. This is great news because regardless of our starting point we are not stuck. We can experience healthy events and make wise choices that will alter our genes in positive ways, bringing healthy benefits and slowing the aging process. Conversely, ongoing unhealthy life events or choices will only add to the damage.

It has been told that the Holy Roman Emperor Fredrick II of Germany wanted to discover the original language spoken by Adam and Eve. He therefore conducted an experiment in which infants were raised by surrogates who were instructed to feed and change the babies but not to hold, cuddle, speak to, or show any affection or ongoing attention to them. The infants were exposed to only the most minimal contact to provide physical nurturance. The hypothesis was that if there was a primal language encoded within humanity, these infants, not influenced by caregivers, would speak it. Would it be Hebrew, Greek, Latin, or something else? The emperor never found out because without touch, without human contact, without interaction, love, and affection—all the infants died.[12]

While Frederick's experiment did not uncover a primal human language, it did reveal the importance of love, affection, human touch, and contact in early childhood. These benefits appear to be important to nonhumans as well. Animal research compared pups born of mothers who regularly licked and groomed them to pups who were neglected by their mothers. Pups without attentive mothers had epigenetic modification of their amygdala (fear circuits) such that they were more anxious and socially impaired than the pups of attentive mothers. What this implied was that the licking and grooming—the affection—was exerting a positive influence on genetic expression and brain development.

However, researchers realized that perhaps the impairments in the amygdala of the neglected pups were genetically programmed to start with and that their mothers were neglectful because they suffered with the same genetic defect. In a follow-up experiment they took the pups born of neglectful mothers and placed them with attentive mothers who licked and groomed them regularly—and the result? Their brains developed normally without any social impairment or increased activity in their anxiety circuits.[13] What this means is that regardless of our starting point at birth our brains remain changeable; early childhood experiences can impact our genetic expression in positive ways and alter brain development.

Yes, childhood is a time of great vulnerability but also great opportunity. Healthy experiences epigenetically alter cellular and brain function in positive ways and lay a foundation for better health and longer life whereas negative experiences do just the opposite.

Child Abuse and Epigenetics

A study of forty-one Canadian men compared the gene expression of twenty-five who were severely abused to sixteen controls. The DNA from their hippocampi (the part of the brain involved in memory, new learning, and calming the stress response) was examined, and 362 epigenetic differences between the two groups were identified. The most significant differences were in genes that coded for neuroplasticity—the ability to change, adapt, and make new neurons and neuron-to-neuron connections. The abuse group had significant impairment in their brains' ability to change and grow when compared to controls.[14]

In another study of over eight hundred people who were followed for thirty-two years, researchers discovered that severe childhood adversity markedly increased the risk of developing depression, diabetes, obesity, and hypercholesterolemia later in life.[15] Multiple other studies document that children who experience severe neglect, physical or sexual abuse, or extreme poverty suffer as adults with higher rates of physical health problems (diabetes mellitus, asthma, obesity, hypercholesterolemia, cardiac disease), mental health problems (depression, anxiety, alcohol and drug problems), and relationship problems and die at a younger age than those who do not experience such childhood adversity.[16] However, research has documented that individuals with trauma histories who participated in cognitive therapy experienced epigenetic changes that brought healing. Specifically, genes associated with the ability to make new neurons (neuroplasticity) were turned on and brain volume increased, and genes associated with calming the brain's stress response were activated. Thus, these individuals were able to experience less emotional and physical stress with improved mental and physical health.[17] This is very good news because regardless of our starting point in life we can make choices that can bring healing, slow aging, and lower our risk of dementia.

Other research has demonstrated the healing power of forgiveness, which is not letting someone off the hook or trusting an abuser or forgetting the past. Forgiveness is resolving the bitterness, resentment, anger, and frustration within oneself. Forgiveness is removing the psychological thorn that causes ongoing emotional pain and chronic activation of the body's stress pathways. In other words, forgiveness heals the one who was wronged; it does not change the one who did wrong. For those who forgive, a history of significant life stress was not a predictor of poor mental health. In women who were abused by their spouses, it was those who not only set boundaries and put an end to the abuse but also forgave who experienced resolution of depression, anxiety, and post-traumatic stress disorder (PTSD) symptoms.[18] Forgiving those who wrong us is healing to us!

Memory and Epigenetics

In an interesting animal study, scientists engineered mice with a specific gene defect that caused memory and learning problems. They divided the mice into two groups (all with the genetic defect). The experimental group was exposed to an "enriched" environment for two weeks during their adolescence. A mouse-enriched environment would be a habitat with climbing apparatus, running wheels, toys, and other interesting textures and shapes. The control group was not exposed to such an enriched environment. It wasn't surprising to the researchers that the mice with the enriched environment had better memory and could learn at a faster rate than the mice without the enriched environment.

What amazed the scientists was what happened to the next generation. The offspring of the control group were born with the genetic defect and grew up with the same memory and learning problems as the parents. But the offspring of the experimental group (mice exposed to an enriched environment) though born with the genetic defect had that defect epigenetically modified such that it did not cause memory and learning problems. These offspring had normal memory and learning even though they did not get an enriched environment during their adolescence. What this means is that the positive experiences in the adolescence of their parents altered the expression of the defective gene in a positive way so that their offspring were born with normal memory and learning.[19]

Regardless of our history we can make choices today that will result in positive health changes to our bodies and brains and thereby slow the aging process and reduce the risk of dementia. The evidence would seem to suggest that if we do this before we have children, not only will we benefit but so will our children and grandchildren. And as we will discover in subsequent chapters, even when healthy changes are implemented late in life they can produce dramatic results to slow, forestall, or even prevent the development of dementia.

▪ LEARNING POINTS ▪

1. We are designed to adapt and change based on our life experiences. Therefore, our choices will either increase or decrease our dementia risk.

2. Essentially every experience in life changes us; we not only form new memories but also our gene expressions and brain structures change, which result in either accelerated or slowed aging.

3. While we cannot change history, we can make modifications in our lives today that will have a positive influence on our gene expression, brain development, health, and aging.

4. Regardless of our starting point in life we can make choices that can bring healing, slow aging, and lower our risk of dementia.

5. Resentment, anger, and bitterness activate the brain's stress pathways, increasing inflammation and accelerating aging while undermining physical and mental health—all of which increase the risk of dementia.

6. Forgiving others who have wronged us calms our internal stress pathways, reducing activation of the immune system, and results in better mental and physical health.

▪ ACTION PLAN: THINGS TO DO ▪

1. Share with friends and family how our life experiences and choices epigenetically change us and that we pass those changes along to future generations.

2. If you have a history of trauma consider cognitive therapy or other specific interventions to address the impact the trauma is having on you today. While you cannot change history, you can change how you react to that history today. Seek interventions that result in reduced activation of your brain's stress circuitry.

3. Evaluate your life history, whether you hold resentment, bitterness, or anger about any wrong done you, and choose to work through it so you can forgive and remove the emotional thorn from your heart. Consider professional therapy if needed.

4. Fill your life with a variety of interesting and engaging activities that stimulate your interest and expand your imagination: art, music, crafts, bird watching, visiting national parks, and so on.

4

Our Genes and Aging

Decay over Time

Bodily decay is gloomy in prospect, but of all human contemplations the most abhorrent is body without mind.

Thomas Jefferson, in a letter to
John Adams, August 1, 1816

A s we discussed earlier, design laws are those protocols, principles, or laws (e.g., laws of health) on which life is constructed to operate. These are the parameters on which reality operates and exists in all domains of life. One of the design laws involved in aging is the Second Law of Thermodynamics, also known as the Law of Entropy, which in layman's terms refers to the fact that if energy isn't put into a system to maintain it and prevent deterioration, the system will slowly decay. Consider walking away from your home or your car and returning twenty years later. If no one did anything to your home or car during the intervening twenty years, in what condition would you find it? It would have decayed. This is a law on how our universe operates: without an influx of energy to maintain order, things slowly become disordered or fall apart—decay.

As we will discuss in chapter 11, our beliefs impact not only our brains but also our physical health, both of which impact aging and the development of dementia. Two grand belief systems, or themes, dominate human thinking—godless evolution and creation by a supreme being (God). Facts, evidence, and life experiences are filtered through these themes. Depending on their underlying belief systems, people draw divergent conclusions when examining the same facts. The purpose of this book is to lead people to healthier lives, which slow the aging process and reduce the risk of dementia. One intervention to accomplish this goal is to identify the design laws (testable parameters) on which life is constructed to operate, to determine which belief system is most consistent with reality (design laws), and to explore whether there are differences in health outcomes based on the belief system held. As we will discover, our beliefs do impact our health and risk of dementia.

The Second Law of Thermodynamics is a testable design law, but what does it have to do with aging and our brains? We can examine the human genome and measure whether the genome is becoming healthier, becoming more complex, and developing enhanced information coding or whether it is slowly decaying, degrading, and deteriorating. Which of the two grand themes, or belief systems, is more consistent with what is actually happening in the human genome and harmonizes with the Second Law of Thermodynamics?

Ancient religious texts describe humanity as originally living in a face-to-face relationship with a Creator God, whose presence was a constant influx of life-sustaining energy. However, when this situation changed and human beings moved out of harmony with their designer, they were told that "dying you will die" (Gen. 2:17 NKJV margin note), meaning if they severed their connection with the source of life-sustaining energy, they would slowly decay and die.

Modern evolutionary theory, taking the opposite view, states that living systems slowly improve, advance, and become more organized with greater complexity *without* any intelligent-energy input. In other words, evolutionary theory states that systems become more ordered, more organized, and more advanced simply by means of random chance causing mutations and natural selection choosing the most advantageous mutations to reproduce. But any scientist can test this theory and recognize quite quickly that without intelligent input of energy, systems decay. What many well-intentioned evolutionary scientists fail to recognize is that when all systems are decaying, selecting the system with the least decay is not the same as advancing or improving the species. Natural selection occurs, to be sure, but what is actually being selected to survive—species with new genetic complexity and advanced organizational health? No! Natural selection can only select from the environment, and all species on earth are decaying. Thus, natural selection selects those specimens that have the least decay, but they are still degraded from previous generations.

John C. Sanford, PhD, an applied geneticist at Cornell University, provides conclusive scientific evidence that the genome of all living creatures, including human beings, is slowly decaying. In his book *Genetic Entropy and the Mystery of the Genome*, Dr. Sanford cites articles, research findings, and publications from across the scientific literature documenting that with every generation multiple new genetic mutations enter the human genome. Further, he documents that there has not been one mutation ever found that improves the species or adds genetic information. In other words, every mutation degrades the species.

For those who are not familiar with genetic science, a simple analogy will help. Dr. Sanford rightly points out that the genome is a microscopic library of information waiting to be accessed and put to use. Consider going to your city's library. The entire library with all its vast information would be analogous to the 3.2 billion molecules found in the twenty-three pairs of chromosomes that make up human DNA. The individual DNA molecules would be all the letters of the alphabet found in the library. Grouping them together they form words. Putting words together forms paragraphs; paragraphs put together form chapters, which would be analogous to individual genes that code for specific products such as hair color, eye color, and the like. The chapters form books, which are analogous to chromosomes, and all the books together (twenty-three pairs of chromosomes) form the library—human DNA.

With this concept in mind, think about what happens if mutations start happening in the books in your library. For example, in one word a single-letter mutation occurs: the word *love* has the *o* replaced by an *i* and now reads as *live*. This is not the original word; the meaning has changed, yet it is still a "readable" word. But the idea or product of this word is different from the original.

This is analogous to single-point mutations in various human genes, which have been documented in the gene that codes for the enzyme that breaks down a critical brain neurotransmitter (dopamine) involved in attention and focus. This mutation results in different functional outcomes.

In the brain, neurons communicate with each other by releasing chemical signals, called *neurotransmitters*, into the spaces between neurons, called *synapses*. Brief puffs of chemicals are released by a neuron that adjacent neurons "see" and respond to. Conceptualize this as being similar to smoke signals. In order to maintain clear communication and prevent "cloudy" and "confused" messages, the brain has multiple mechanisms to clear the synaptic sky between signals. Just imagine how difficult it would be to read smoke signals if the smoke never dissipated between signals.

One mechanism the brain uses to remove neurotransmitters from the synaptic spaces are reuptake pumps that work like little vacuum cleaners to pull the transmitter back into the releasing cell to repackage and reuse for more signaling later. But these pumps don't get 100 percent of the neurotransmitter, so the brain has enzymes in the synaptic spaces to break down and remove residual neurotransmitters. One of these enzymes is catechol-O-methyltransferase (COMT), and it breaks down the neurotransmitter dopamine. The *COMT* gene that produces this enzyme is located on chromosome 22. But this gene has had a single-point mutation (one letter has been replaced with another, but it can still be read). Therefore, two genetic forms of the gene can be found: one form with the amino acid valine (Val) at position 108 on the gene; the other with the amino acid methionine (Met) at position 108.

Because of this mutation, the COMT enzyme in individuals with Val instead of Met is more active at body temperature—so active, in fact, it is clearing the dopamine (signal) before it can even be registered. This would be analogous to trying to give smoke signals in high winds; the wind is clearing the smoke so fast no message can be sent. As a result these individuals will have less dopamine available. Signaling between neurons is undermined by this very active form of the enzyme. Memory testing has documented that persons with the Val "letter" in the *COMT* gene perform worse on short-term memory testing than those with the Met "letter."[1]

But our library of information has other more complex products that require more than just single words; they require full sentences. Sometimes mutations occur in which, instead of replacing a single letter, an entire word is deleted or replaced. Imagine reading a sentence that is missing a word. If it is a critical word the meaning may be completely wrong. Your instruction manual should read: "Do not connect the green and red wires." But your manual is missing the word "not" and reads: "Do connect the green and red wires." The outcome could be devastating.

Worse still are mutations in which entire sentences (genes) are deleted. In such cases the information simply isn't there for the body to produce what is needed. An example of this type of mutation is Prader-Willi syndrome, in which seven genes on chromosome

15 are deleted. Fortunately, this disorder is rare, but because such a vast amount of information is lost it is quite severe, and those with it have poor muscle tone, impaired cognitive and sexual development, behavior problems, and often insatiable hunger that leads to obesity.[2]

Another type of mutation includes repeats in which a gene, or portion thereof, repeats itself multiple times. Consider a book in which one word word word word word word word repeats itself many times. Huntington's disease is caused by a short three-nucleotide (letter) repeat that occurs multiple times. The gene where this repeat occurs is found on chromosome 4 and produces a protein called *huntingtin*. The precise function of huntingtin is unclear, but it is important for development and is highly expressed in neurons. When more than thirty-six of these repeats occur, a protein that is toxic to neurons is produced with the sad result manifesting in Huntington's disease.[3]

There are also transposons, which are sometimes called *jumping genes*, in which a gene will move from its proper place to a new location on the chromosome.[4] This would be like having a sentence in a book randomly moved to some other place in the book. The impact is widely variable depending on which gene is involved and where it moves.

You can imagine how difficult it would be if you had an instruction manual on how to build an engine, but in the manual there were misspelled words, missing words and sentences, sections with long repeats, and instances where words or sentences were moved from their proper place to random new locations within the manual.

With every human generation more of these mutations occur. This means that the human genome is slowly decaying. Here are the estimated new mutations occurring *per generation*:

- Mitochondrial—less than 1 percent
- Nucleotide substitution—100–300

- Satellite mutations—100–300
- Deletions—2–6 percent or more
- Duplications/insertions—2–6 percent or more
- Inversions/translocations—too numerous to count
- Conversions—probably thousands
- Total per person per generation—*greater than 1,000 new mutations*[5]

Evolutionary scientists will argue that mutations allow for advantages in certain toxic situations and thus, with an extremely narrow view, argue that such mutations are beneficial and advance the species. A classic example is sickle cell anemia. This condition occurs because of a single-nucleotide polymorphism (one-letter-in-one-word replacement) in the gene that codes for hemoglobin. Hemoglobin is the protein that carries oxygen in the blood. The mutation causes the shape of red blood cells to deform from their smooth, disc-like shapes to ragged, sickle-like shapes.

Because we have two sets of genes, one set from mother and one set from father, a person can have two good genes, one good and one bad gene, or two bad genes. Only those with two bad genes develop full-blown sickle cell anemia. Because those with one copy of the bad gene have been noted to be resistant to malaria, and thereby more likely to survive in malaria-infested areas than those with two good genes, evolutionary biologists often point to this mutation as evidence of how evolution advances the species.

This is a beautiful example of missing the forest for the trees—missing the larger reality by focusing on a less-significant fact. It is true that those with one copy of the bad sickle cell gene are more likely to survive in malaria-ridden environments. Thus, they are more likely to pass their genes along and thereby continue the existence of this mutation. However, this mutation does *not* add information to the human genome, nor does it result in stronger and healthier humans with greater life expectancy. Further, this single mutation, which confers advantage in surviving malaria, does not prevent the multiplicity of other damaging DNA mutations from occurring with every generation. So regardless of whether one survives malaria, their genome has been degraded by a minimum of one thousand new damaging mutations. Does natural selection occur? Absolutely, but what evolutionary biologists remain blinded to is that every genetic option is degrading, regardless of which individual is selected to survive! At age sixty-five a person will have six thousand point mutations in their DNA that were not there when they were born. The human genome is slowly decaying, and this decay is one factor in aging.

Genetic Mutation and Aging

While genetic mutations can happen spontaneously, there are many environmental factors that cause mutations and thus cause genetic decay and accelerate aging. To the degree we can avoid or reduce exposure to these factors, we can slow the aging process and reduce our risk of dementia. Environmental factors that cause mutations are called *mutagens*, and they can be physical, chemical, or biological.

Physical mutagens are ionizing radiation such as gamma and alpha particles and X-rays. These particles physically damage the DNA, causing mutations. The most common sources are Cobalt-60 and Cesium-137. Cobalt-60 is a by-product of nuclear reactors and is used in medical radiation therapy, to irradiate food in order to kill pests, and in some industrial applications. Cesium-137 is also a by-product of nuclear reactors and can be used in medical radiation therapy and some industrial applications. Obviously, we would want to avoid exposure to such particles. Get X-rays only when medically necessary. If working in the medical field and exposed to X-ray equipment, always wear lead aprons and other protective equipment. If working with medical radioactive material, always follow handling procedures and wear radiation detectors.

The other major source of physical mutagens is ultraviolet radiation, which is in sunlight and is a major contributing factor to skin cancers. It is this wavelength of light that sunscreens are designed to block. In regard to aging most of us have seen individuals who have had excessive sun exposure throughout life; their skin is more damaged and aged than that of persons with less sun exposure. That is because of the greater damage occurring to the DNA (and other molecules) in their skin cells, which accelerates decay and aging. We can reduce risk by limiting sun exposure and by using sunscreen when in the sun.

Chemical mutagens, which are chemicals that can mutate our DNA, include reactive oxygen species (ROS) (which we will explore in detail in a later chapter) and polycyclic aromatic hydrocarbons (PAH). PAH can be found in abundance in fossil fuels (oil and coal), meat cooked at high temperatures such as grilling and charring, and tobacco smoke.[6] These PAH molecules have been shown to increase various types of cancer.[7] They can also alter genetic expression and brain development in children and increase cognitive and behavior problems in children whose mothers breathed high amounts of PAH (air pollution from burning fossil fuels) while pregnant with them.[8] Other chemical mutagens include arsenic, cadmium, chromium, and nickel.[9] Keeping our environment clean, reducing air pollution, avoiding tobacco smoke, and not eating meats charred or grilled will reduce exposure to these damaging compounds and thereby slow aging and reduce both cancer and dementia risk.

Biological mutagens include certain viruses and bacteria, as well as the transposons we discussed earlier. One example of this is the human papillomavirus (HPV), which is sexually transmitted and known to cause a variety of cancers. HPV infection causes a cascade of responses in the body, resulting in gene mutations that contribute to various cancers, such as cervical cancer.[10] Fortunately, vaccines are now available to prevent HPV infection.

Telomeres and Aging

As we wind up our chapter on human genetics and aging, we need to discuss telomeres and aging. Telomeres are critical in cellular replication. As cells are damaged or just wear out with age, they need to be replaced. The way the body does this is by one cell copying itself to make another or by progenitor cells (factory cells) making new cells. But in order for the new cell to have all the abilities and functionality of the parent cell, it needs its own copy of the library of information (chromosomes). When a cell divides (mitosis), it copies its chromosomes so that both cells will have a complete set of genetic information. The telomeres are the end caps on each chromosome. Consider them like the plastic caps on your shoelaces. They keep the genetic material together and organized and prevent unraveling. But the length of these end caps is critical in determining the ability of the cell to replicate. If they get too short the cell can no longer copy itself or make new cells.

In the 1970s it was discovered that when cells replicated, the telomere end caps didn't fully replicate. In fact, they shortened with each replication. If the telomeres get too short the cell can no longer divide. If cells can't divide, they can't replace damaged and worn-out cells and thus aging occurs. The results are readily seen when one compares the skin of an elderly person with that of a child. If both experience a similar superficial cut the child will heal quickly, but the older person's skin will struggle to heal. One factor is that the shorter telomeres in the elderly person make it harder for their cells to reproduce and close the wound.

The telomeres of an infant contain approximately eight thousand base pairs. By age thirty-five the telomeres contain thirty-five hundred base pairs and by age sixty-five, only fifteen hundred.[11] Recent research has documented that individuals with mood disorders as well as children who have been institutionalized have shorter telomeres than healthy control subjects. Further, hostility and negative emotions can shorten telomeres.

Scientists have recently documented that telomere length may be able to predict remaining life span. Lawrence Honig, MD, PhD, a professor of neurology at Columbia University, and his colleagues studied 1,978 people ranging from 66 to 101 years of age, with the average age of 78, from multiethnic backgrounds (African American, Hispanic, and white). They discovered that men in general had shorter telomeres than women, those with shorter telomeres died at an earlier age, and shorter telomeres were associated with developing Alzheimer's dementia.[12] However, men do not appear to have shorter telomeres at birth; instead, their telomeres shorten more rapidly throughout life.[13] This suggests that the modifiable factors listed below are likely playing a significant role in the gender differences seen later in life. Interestingly, researchers also noted a wide range of telomere lengths across the age range, meaning age itself didn't predict the length of one's telomeres but telomere length did predict how much longer one could expect to live.

One factor that did impact telomere length was paternal age (age of the father) at the time of conception; the older the father at the time of conception the longer the telomeres in his children, both sons and daughters. Older age of the mother had either no impact or a negative effect on telomere length. The longer telomeres also seemed to pass down to the grandchildren of the older father—and if the son was older when his children were conceived this added further lengthening effects to his children's telomeres.[14] And the longer telomeres at birth did translate to living longer lives.[15] What seems to be happening is that genetics accounts for about 80 percent of telomere length and environment affects about 20 percent of telomere length.

Factors that have been noted to accelerate the shortening of telomeres include childhood adversity,[16] mood disorders, relationship conflicts and negative mental attitudes, and hostility. Factors that have been associated with lengthening telomeres include plant-based diet, stress reduction and meditation, and physical exercise.[17] Therefore, interventions that bring conflict resolution, resolve internal stress (such as forgiving those who have wronged us), and allow avoidance of activities that increase stress (cheating on one's spouse, embezzling from an employer, falsifying an insurance claim, etc.) will have a positive impact on telomere length—as well as reduce many other damaging stress-related processes within the body. Additionally, our worldview impacts our mental stress level. As we will document in later chapters, stress reduction and meditation are directly connected to our belief systems. Belief systems that enhance reasoning, thinking, and evaluation of evidence and that include a benevolent God are the healthiest. Belief systems with no God but that promote reasoning, thinking, evaluation of evidence, and a benevolent mindset toward others are the next healthiest. But belief systems with authoritarian gods that undermine thinking, reasoning, and evaluation of evidence and incite fear by focusing on rule keeping and punishment for rule breaking are unhealthy, accelerate aging, and increase the risk of dementia. Thus, our worldview is directly connected to our life practices, stress management, and mode of relating to others and can contribute to both aging and dementia risk. We will explore specific reasons and evidences for this in later chapters. At this point, my goal is for the reader to be willing to think, evaluate evidence, and consider different viewpoints but only make a change in belief when fully persuaded by the weight of evidence.

As was mentioned, one factor that lengthens telomeres is a healthy diet. A recent study of more than thirty-six hundred adults found that doubling the amount of carotenoids (antioxidant molecules that give plants color) in the diet lengthened telomeres 2 percent. And those in the study with the highest levels of carotenoids had telomeres 5–8 percent longer![18] Foods high in carotenoids include carrots, sweet potatoes, tomatoes, and green leafy vegetables. Not surprisingly, a study by Dean Ornish published in *Lancet Oncology* in 2013 found that a lifestyle change to a plant-based diet resulted in increased activity in telomerase (the enzyme that lengthens telomeres).[19]

One study on exercise and telomere length found slightly contradictory results. It found that not all exercise lengthened telomeres, but standing several hours a day did. Another way to interpret the data is that long-term sitting or a significantly sedentary lifestyle shortens telomeres.[20]

Clearly, telomere length is involved in cellular reproduction and thereby the ability to maintain youth and vitality. But unrestrained telomere lengthening is not the answer. At least one study has documented that many human cancers occur because of unrestrained telomere lengthening, which results in unregulated cellular reproduction—that is, cancer.[21]

Our goal, then, is not unregulated telomere growth but to make lifestyle choices that reduce or delay telomere shortening and promote telomere health and length. It is striking to note that the Bible is not only more consistent with the science of genetic entropy but also connects relationship health and childhood peace with longer life (Exod. 20:12)—something science has now proven to be true.

▪ LEARNING POINTS ▪

1. Without energy, input systems decay over time.
2. The human genome is slowly decaying.
3. Environmental factors can damage our genome and accelerate aging; these include radiation, pollutants, and infections.
4. Telomeres are the end caps that enable cells to divide and replicate. If they get too short, cells can no longer divide, impairing our body's ability to heal or replace worn-out cells and thus contributing to aging.
5. Telomeres are shortened by chronic stress, conflict, a sedentary lifestyle, and a diet devoid of fruits and vegetables.

6. Telomeres are lengthened by physical activity, foods high in carotenoids, conflict resolution, and stress management.

7. Our worldview (belief system) impacts how we interpret facts, the lifestyle choices we make, our mode and method of relating, and ultimately how we manage stress and conflict resolution, thus impacting aging.

▪ ACTION PLAN: THINGS TO DO ▪

1. Avoid sources of radiation: get X-rays only when needed; use sunscreen, hats, and other protective measures; if working in medical or industrial fields that utilize radioactive material, be vigilant with radiation detectors and use proper shielding.

2. Reduce eating meat and meat cooked at high temperatures; when cooking meat, cook at lower temperatures.

3. Increase plant-based food options (carrots, sweet potatoes, tomatoes, green leafy vegetables).

4. Avoid environments with high amounts of air pollution.

5. Avoid tobacco smoke, including secondhand smoke.

6. Consider getting the HPV vaccine.

7. Reduce the risk of sexually transmitted mutagens by committing to sexual abstinence before marriage and monogamy after marriage.

8. Be physically active in life; avoid a sedentary lifestyle.

9. Resolve relationship conflicts and reduce resentment and hostility.

10. Think for yourself, evaluate evidence, and consider which worldview is not only most consistent with the evidence but also harmonizes with design law and promotes the greatest health.

PART 2

OXIDATIVE STRESS AND AGING

5

Obesity and Aging

The Link Is Unmistakable

> Tell people that biology and the environment cause obesity and they are offered the one thing we have to avoid: an excuse.
>
> Andrew Lansley, British Secretary of State for Health[1]

Aging—the slow decline in vitality and ability—affects us all. Yet while people move through time at a constant rate, not everyone ages at the same rate during the same amount of time lived. Some individuals deteriorate (age) much faster than others. While we cannot affect the passage of time, we can affect our passage through time—we can make intelligent choices to maximize health and slow the decay so that we grow older with greater vitality and retained abilities.

When we know what accelerates aging, we can make intelligent choices to minimize or avoid harmful factors and embrace actions that promote vitality and youthfulness. So what factors accelerate aging and loss of vitality, and what actions can we take to maintain our abilities to the highest extent possible?

One of the major factors in accelerated aging is oxidative stress, which is the damage to DNA, proteins, lipids, and other body tissues caused by oxygen-containing molecules. Cut an apple and leave it on the counter for an hour and what happens? It browns; this is oxidation—oxygen molecules binding with and damaging the fruit. Oxidation damages the body's tissues and accelerates aging. This is why we hear so much about antioxidants—factors that scavenge the oxidizing molecules and protect us from oxidative damage.

Inflammation

In this book I use the term *inflammation* or *inflammatory cascade* when describing various factors that accelerate aging. In fact, it is through the inflammatory pathway of the body that most of the negative health factors cause accelerated aging and increase our risk of dementia. Whatever increases inflammation will accelerate aging and raise dementia risk, while whatever decreases inflammation will slow aging and lower dementia risk.

So what do I mean by inflammation?

Inflammation is when the body responds to attacks (either by injury, infection, or disease) by mobilizing its forces to neutralize and resolve the attack, thus restoring the body to normal function. The body's inflammatory response is exquisitely complex with many cells (white blood cells—neutrophils, monocytes, eosinophils, mast cells), proteins, and other factors (chemokines, cytokines, adhesion molecules, oxygen-containing molecules, etc.) working in orchestrated cascades to resolve threats, bring healing, and restore normal function. We have all experienced this when we have had a cold or some other infection. These inflammatory factors, which are designed to neutralize threats to the body, impact the body in other ways as well and cause symptoms such as malaise, fatigue, concentration problems, loss of appetite, and achiness—symptoms we often experience when fighting a sickness. When all things go as designed such inflammation is limited to the level of the threat and resolves when the injury is healed or the infection cleared.

However, sometimes things go wrong and the body's inflammatory system stays turned on. This can happen in the aftermath of an infection or injury and can contribute to chronic fatigue, autoimmune disorders, and chronic pain states. The body can also turn on this inflammatory cascade in response to certain foods, toxins, pollutants, or other ingested substances as we shall soon discover.

Finally, the body can also gear up its inflammatory response in reaction to *perceived* threats. This means chronic anxiety, worry, conflict, and stress can turn on this system and increase within the body the concentration of circulating molecules that are designed to damage (oxidize) invading viruses and bacteria. But when we are under chronic worry and stress, the concentration of these molecules increases without any foreign invaders for them to attack. So instead they begin damaging healthy cells within our bodies. This is inflammation—elevation and activation of immune cells, chemokines, cytokines, adhesion molecules, and oxygen-containing molecules—which causes widespread problems in our bodies, including accelerated aging, and, as we will see in chapter 14, directly contributes to the development of dementia.

So what are the factors that increase oxidative damage to our brains? In Part 2 we will explore three factors that increase oxidation and accelerate aging—obesity, sugar, and toxic substances.

Obesity

Perhaps the most significant factor that increases oxidative damage to our bodies and accelerates aging is obesity! Excessive fat tissue produces reactive oxygen species (ROS), which are molecules that contain oxygen capable of interacting with our body tissues and causing damage. Further, excess fat reduces the body's antioxidant enzymes, undermining our body's ability to eliminate these toxic molecules.[2] Obesity increases oxidative stress.[3]

At age seventy an obese person's brain has 8 percent less brain volume and appears sixteen years older than a normal-weight person's brain of the same age. Also, at age seventy an overweight person's brain has 4 percent less brain volume and appears eight years older than a normal-weight person's brain of the same age.[4]

Obesity in America is rampant: more than 40 percent of men and 42 percent of women between the ages of fifty-five and sixty-four are obese; between ages sixty-five and seventy-four, over 36 percent of men and 35 percent of women are obese. That is well more than one in three. If we include those who are overweight, the numbers are staggering: after age fifty-five approximately 80 percent of men and 70 percent of women are either overweight or obese![5]

Historically, people viewed obesity as a simple matter of calories consumed versus calories burned—if people ate more calories than they burned, they got obese. While this is true as the final common denominator, many factors other than the amount of food ingested impact the body's energy balance. In other words, obesity is quite complex with a multiplicity of factors contributing to alterations in the body's ability to absorb and utilize energy.

Sleep and Obesity

Studies have shown that sleep deprivation can alter the body's hormones that impact metabolism, thus altering its ability to burn energy reserves (fat) and increasing the risk of obesity.[6] According to the Centers for Disease Control (CDC), fifty to seventy million Americans have some type of sleep disorder.[7] A 2009 multistate

CDC survey of over seventy thousand adults found that more than 35 percent of people slept fewer than seven hours per night.[8] And according to a Sleep in America Poll conducted on behalf of the National Sleep Foundation, approximately 20 percent of Americans get fewer than six hours of sleep per night.[9] Sleep deprivation is a serious problem and alters normal body energy use, contributing to obesity, which contributes to increased oxidative stress. In chapter 9 we will explore in greater detail the importance of sleep for healthy brain function and factors that interfere with normal sleep.

Soybeans and Obesity

Over the last one hundred years dietary patterns in many westernized countries have changed. In the United States there has been a significant shift in the percentages of dietary oils ingested—away from healthy oils to more obesity-promoting fats. Historically, the human diet contained no more than 1 percent of the oil linoleic acid (LA), which is an omega-6 fatty acid found in a variety of foods but highly concentrated in soybean oil. Over the past century the United States' dietary intake of LA has increased from 1 percent to 8 percent of daily caloric intake. Soybean oil is used in most margarines and shortenings as well as in mayonnaise, salad dressing, frozen foods, imitation dairy, various meat products, and commercial baking goods.

Recent research has demonstrated that LA is a precursor to two brain-derived marijuana-like compounds called *endocannabinoids*. These compounds are active in the brain region that controls appetite, caloric intake, and satiety. Increasing activity in this brain region triggers increased appetite and is associated with increasing obesity.[10]

Remarkably, in animal studies conducted to evaluate the impact of increasing LA in the diet, animals fed diets composed of

35 percent fat and 8 percent LA had significantly greater obesity than animals fed 60 percent fat diets and only 1 percent LA. This indicates that the LA trigger of endocannabinoid receptors mediates obesity. Even if one lowers the amount of total fat in the diet, if the diet retains a high percentage of LA, obesity risk increases.

However, supplementing the 8 percent LA diet with 1 percent omega-3 fatty acids from fish oil (eicosapentaenoic acid [EPA] and docosahexaenoic acid [DHA]) reversed the elevations of endocannabinoids and decreased both food consumption and obesity.

Further, insulin levels were not altered in either group, meaning the obesity was occurring before diabetic metabolic dysregulation occurred and was not caused by insulin resistance or driven by carbohydrate intake.

Soybean oil (not to be confused with soybean protein) is about 50 percent LA by weight and is the single greatest contributor to the increase in LA in the American diet over the last century. Combine this increased consumption of LA with the reduction in EPA and DHA through either less fish consumed or increased farm-raised fish (which are generally devoid of EPA and DHA), and we have a dietary setup for increased obesity. This dietary change corresponds with the increased prevalence of obesity seen in the United States.

A diet low in EPA and DHA and high in LA is associated with not only increased obesity but also increased risk for mental health–related problems, including psychosis, mood disorders, and dementia.[11] Therefore, reducing LA, primarily by reducing soy intake and increasing EPA and DHA in the diet, has been shown to be healthy for the brain. Other sources of LA include safflower, sunflower, and sesame oil, as well as Brazil nuts and pine nuts. Alternative oils low in LA include canola (21 percent), olive (10 percent), palm (10 percent), and coconut (2 percent).

Foods high in omega-3s (EPA and DHA) include wild sardines, salmon, mackerel, tuna, and trout. Freshwater fish have significantly less EPA and DHA than cold-water ocean fish. EPA and

DHA are not produced in plants, with the exception of some sea algae and seaweed. Therefore, vegans are encouraged to find a seaweed supplement high in EPA and DHA. Flax seed is high in omega-3 (ALA) but is poorly converted in the body to the form the brain needs, with approximately 8 percent converted to EPA and less than 1 percent converted to DHA. Therefore, flax seed supplement is not recommended as a substitute for EPA and DHA.[12]

Genetically Modified Foods and Obesity

Another factor impacting obesity rates today may be genetically modified foods. I first became concerned about genetically modified foods when studies began to emerge demonstrating that we are impacted not only by the fats, proteins, and carbohydrates of the foods we eat but also by the genetic material of consumed foods. Whatever food we eat contains the DNA and RNA of that plant or animal, and its genetic material is also absorbed into our bodies. Science now demonstrates that ingested genetic material can alter how our genes are expressed. One study found that small pieces of RNA from ingested rice alter the human gene that codes for how LDL cholesterol is processed.[13] This means the genetic material from the foods we eat can alter how our genes are expressed.

With this thought in mind, I became troubled by the amount of genetically modified food in our food supply and the serious lack of evidence demonstrating that it is safe and does not cause genetic modifications damaging to our health. A recent animal study in Norway lends support to my concern. Rats that were fed genetically modified food grew fatter than rats fed nongenetically modified food. This occurred whether the rats ate the genetically modified corn directly or ate fish that were fed genetically modified corn. Professor Åshild Krogdahl of the Norwegian School of Veterinary Science rightly asks, "If the same effect applies to humans, how would it impact on people eating this type of corn over a number of years, or even eating meat from animals feeding on this corn?"[14] While the exact reasons for these differences in weight have not been determined, altered gene expression is one possibility.

Until much more research is done to prove the health safety of genetically modified foods, the wisest course of action is to select organic, non-GMO foods whenever possible. This may be difficult to achieve in the United States where as much as 75 percent of the food in supermarkets contains genetically modified ingredients. The law passed in 2016 requiring the labeling of GMO-containing foods allows manufacturers to comply by placing a QR code on the packaging that, when scanned by a smartphone, would take the consumer to a website informing them of the GMO content. I would encourage those concerned to speak with your supermarket managers and request they do this research and clearly label items for sale in their stores as GMO-free items.

Gut Bacteria and Obesity

Other research has documented that obese people and thin people have different types of bacteria living in their stomachs and intestines, and these differences can contribute to obesity.[15] Obese people had fewer bacteria called Bacteroidetes and greater amounts of Firmicutes as compared to lean people.[16] Further research demonstrated that diet impacts the balance of microbes living in our guts. When dietary changes were made that resulted in weight loss, Bacteroidetes increased and Firmicutes decreased in the gut.[17] Typically, fiber in plants is indigestible to humans, which means the energy in such material (like cellulose) is not absorbed by humans and doesn't contribute to caloric intake. However, studies have demonstrated that bacteria living in the gut can metabolize fiber and contribute as much as 10 percent of daily caloric intake. This may be why some obese people don't lose weight even when eating foods low in calories but high in fiber.[18] This means that addressing obesity isn't as simple as merely calculating the number of calories consumed versus those burned but includes the impact that the bacteria living in one's bowels are having. Are the gut bacteria converting typically inaccessible consumed calories (cellulose) into absorbable calories? The evidence strongly suggests the answer is yes.

Our food choices do change the gut flora and these changes occur quickly. One recent study found that people on a plant-based diet who began eating animal products (eggs, milk, cheese, meat) experienced changes in gut bacteria within one day.[19] And the bacterial changes with the animal-based diet were associated with greater risk for inflammatory diseases.[20] Foods high in plant fiber (legumes, fruit, broccoli, etc.) increase the growth in good bacteria that promote weight loss, whereas foods high in sugar and animal fats promote bacteria that increase inflammation and oxidation.[21] Interestingly, this may be one of the reasons gastric bypass surgery often results in weight loss. Studies have shown that one factor in the weight loss associated with gastric bypass surgery is not simply a reduction in calories consumed but also the marked change in gut flora that the surgery triggers.[22]

The bottom line on obesity in this regard is that it isn't just the total calories consumed that matters but also the types of foods consumed, which alter gut bacteria. Animal-based foods increase the bacteria that contributes to obesity, whereas plant-based foods that are high in fiber increase the bacteria that promotes weight loss. Reducing animal products and increasing plant-based food choices is one action you can take to reduce obesity risk.

Not All Body Fat Is Equal

The body has two populations of adipose, or fat: white and brown. White fat is associated with obesity and is very difficult to mobilize and remove from our bodies. Brown fat is involved in regulating body temperature and thus actively burns calories. While white fat cells contain only fat, brown fat cells in addition to the fat also contain iron-rich mitochondria and more capillaries to provide oxygen for energy use. As we age, we tend to lose brown fat from our bodies; this may contribute to the midlife spread, the typical increase in body fat that happens in our fifties. Recent research has demonstrated that diet, gut bacteria, and inflammation and the immune response to it directly impact the amount of brown fat in our bodies and thus whether we are obese or remain thin throughout life.

Researchers at Harvard and Conway Institute at University College Dublin have demonstrated that an immune cell, invariant natural killer T (iNKT), is integral in activating the small protein fibroblast growth factor-21 (FGF-21). This protein, when available, triggers the body to convert white fat into brown fat and results in increased energy production from the fat cells, which raises body temperature and basic metabolic rate and brings about significant weight loss. Blood samples from obese individuals showed reduced iNKT cells. But obese individuals who lost weight after bariatric surgery showed increased iNKT cells. Similarly, in animal studies when the animals were placed on a high-fat diet, they lost their iNKT cells and gained weight, but when the diet was returned to normal the iNKT cells increased and weight loss occurred. When iNKT cells were removed from normal mice and injected into obese iNKT-deficient mice, the obese mice lost weight, had improved insulin sensitivity, and improved triglycerides—all indicators of improvement in metabolic profile. Finally, the researchers tested a lipid (alpha-galactosylceramide [aGC]) known to activate the iNKT cells and discovered that a single dose of this lipid resulted in reversal of diabetes, marked weight loss, and lowering of blood lipid levels.[23] Though not currently available as a treatment, hopefully it soon will be.

What is interesting is that as people become obese, the iNKT cells are lost and the ability to produce brown fat is reduced.

Contributing factors to the reduction of the iNKT cells are diets high in fat and sugars and low in dietary fiber, the Western diet. One potential mechanism for this was recently discovered and has to do with the bacteria living in our gut. As we just discussed, the bacteria living in our gut can impact our caloric absorption. But recent research has demonstrated that one type of bacteria, *Bacteroides*, also produces the glycosphingolipid α-galactosylceramide (α-GalCer$_{Bf}$), which is structurally related to aGC and has been shown to be an activator of our iNKT cells in both *vitro* and *vivo* studies.[24] This means that a plant-based diet rich in fiber and low in animal fats will cause growth of good bacteria (*Bacteroides*), which produce a protein that will activate our iNKT cells, which in turn will produce a protein that will trigger white fat to turn to brown fat—increasing our metabolism, burning fat, and reducing obesity.

Genetic Expression and Obesity

On a similar note, as we discussed in chapter 2, research has found that during fetal development environmental factors can impact gene expression that regulates how efficiently one absorbs energy from food. During WWII in the Netherlands there was a severe food shortage. People averaged about five hundred calories of food intake per day, including pregnant women.

Children born to women during this food shortage grew up with higher rates of obesity, diabetes mellitus, and metabolic problems than their siblings born to the same parents when food was more plentiful. Researchers have identified that the severe food shortage altered the expression of a specific gene (*IGF2*) associated with energy absorption from food. This particular gene was altered in a way that caused increased expression and resulted in what scientists believe is the ability of these individuals to extract more calories from the same food as compared to others where this gene is less active.[25]

For some, then, obesity has little to do with their lifestyle or food choices but with the epigenetics governing metabolism genes. Understanding this may provide psychological relief and reduce guilt, blame, and shame cycles, which only activate stress pathways and thus contribute to increased inflammation and undermine the ability to lose weight. Additionally, persons who may be obese due to such epigenetic changes may have tried various diet or lifestyle programs with minimal results and have become discouraged and given up—thinking, *Why bother?*—and resigned themselves to eating whatever they want. This would be a terrible mistake because it isn't just obesity itself that is the problem but also the increased inflammation throughout the body that causes the negative brain changes. Lifestyle choices that reduce inflammation will reduce the damage and add protection to the brain—even if the person remains overweight.

Therefore, if you are struggling with excessive body fat and have tried lifestyle changes to lose weight but have experienced only limited success, don't fall into the trap of believing that your choices don't matter—they do! Choosing to make healthy lifestyle choices, including walking daily (see chap. 8), regular, normal sleep cycles (see chap. 9), anti-inflammatory diet (see chap. 6), mental rest and relaxation (see chap. 10), and formulating healthy belief systems (see chap. 11), will reduce inflammatory stress, improve brain function and cognitive performance, and reduce dementia risk *even if the total body weight doesn't change!*

Infections and Obesity

Another factor that can increase inflammation is infections, and certain viral infections have been shown to contribute to obesity. Adenoviruses are a family of viruses that infect humans, causing the common cold and stomach, eye, and bladder infections. One particular adenovirus (Ad-36) has been shown to cause obesity in humans.[26] The exact mechanism is unknown but is potentially related to increased inflammation.

Inflammation and Obesity

Finally, inflammation causes insulin resistance, which results in the body increasing the amount of insulin circulating in the blood. Insulin not only regulates the body's glucose levels but also signals fat cells to create more fat and to stop adipose cells from breaking down stored fat to be burned off. In order to burn stored fat rather than create more fat, the signal sent by insulin to fat cells must be reduced. An interesting animal study revealed that knocking out the insulin receptor in fat cells resulted in the animals losing up to 70 percent of their body fat in three months, despite eating 55 percent more food per gram of body weight—and they lived 18 percent longer than animals without the insulin receptor knocked out.[27] The weight-loss strategy of lowering insulin is the core principle behind the various high-fat, low-carb weight-loss programs. If one reduces carbs, then one reduces the production of insulin and thereby promotes weight loss. Such diets focus exclusively on weight loss, not on aging and slowing the loss of vitality and retaining abilities. So while it is true that reducing obesity is beneficial to slowing aging, one can still have accelerated aging with a normal body weight if inflammation is not reduced. A highly inflammatory diet with normal body weight is not the best approach to slowing the aging process.

Anything that increases inflammation will contribute to insulin resistance and promote obesity. Highly processed foods, junk food, and fast food contribute to obesity not only because of the high concentration of calories but also because these foods are highly inflammatory foods. Thus, they increase glucose while simultaneously contributing to insulin resistance. And of course, once obesity occurs the adipose tissue itself creates inflammatory factors, contributing to further insulin resistance and increasing production of fat stores—a downward spiral.

While excessive body fat increases production of oxidizing molecules and reduces the antioxidant enzymes in the body, it isn't merely the body fat itself but also the constellation of other lifestyle factors that typically accompany and contribute to obesity that are the real problem when it comes to aging. Obese people generally don't exercise as much as thin people, thereby reducing exercise-induced neurotrophins (proteins that act like fertilizer in the brain to keep neurons healthy and increase the production of new neurons and neuron-to-neuron connections, which improve learning and slow cognitive decline). Also, those with excessive body fat typically eat unhealthier diets, with foods that are inflammatory in nature, and often have sleep problems, which accelerate cognitive decline.

The point of all of this is that obese individuals have accelerated brain decline and increased risks of dementia because of multiple negative factors working together. Even if one doesn't lose weight but addresses the other negative factors, the damaging toll on the brain will be reduced. Therefore, an obese person who gets normal sleep, walks thirty minutes daily, eats a healthy anti-inflammatory diet, gets regular mental rest, and manages life stress well will reduce the negative impact of obesity on their brains, slow cognitive decline, and have better memory and cognitive performance.

▪ LEARNING POINTS ▪

1. Oxidative stress accelerates aging and has multiple causes.
2. Inflammation is the activation of cells and molecules within the body that increases oxidation and can be caused by injury, infection, toxins, foods, and unremitting mental stress.
3. Obesity is one cause of oxidative stress.

4. Obesity is complex and is caused by more than just calories consumed and calories burned; it also involves the type of food ingested, which alters gut flora, impacting immune response and altering the brown-to-white-fat ratio.

5. Increasing omega-3 fatty acids and reducing LA, getting regular nightly sleep, reducing inflammatory foods, increasing physical activity, and perhaps avoiding genetically modified foods can move the energy balance away from storage to utilization with reduction in obesity, thereby reducing oxidative stress and slowing the aging process.

6. For some individuals epigenetic changes increase their energy absorption from food, contributing to obesity with typically normal food intake.

7. It isn't merely excessive body fat that contributes to brain volume loss and accelerated dementia risk but also the constellation of other factors that increase inflammation. Reducing these other factors reduces dementia risk and improves cognitive performance, even if total body fat doesn't change.

▪ ACTION PLAN: THINGS TO DO ▪

1. Reduce soybean (and other high LA) oil in the diet.

2. Use olive oil or other low LA oils more frequently.

3. Increase daily intake of omega-3 fatty acids (DHA and EPA).

4. Ensure regular nightly sleep of seven to eight hours for adults.

5. Move toward a plant-based diet, rich in fiber and low in animal fats, which will cause growth of good bacteria in the gut.

6. Consider reducing GMO foods.

7. Avoid guilt, shame, and blame cycles if making healthy life choices but still remain overweight.

8. Walk twenty to thirty minutes each day.

6

Sugar, Oxidation, and Aging

We Are What We Eat

Sugar Is the New Tobacco, so Let's Treat It
That Way

headline in *Medscape Psychiatry*,
October 31, 2016

W ho doesn't like a sweet treat—some candy, cake, ice
cream, or pie? Many of today's seniors remember
Shirley Temple singing, "The Good Ship Lollipop,"
"a sweet trip to the candy shop"; crackerjacks, peppermint, tootsie
rolls, devil's food cake, and if you eat too much "you'll awake with
a tummy ache."

But the sad truth is that sugar has done far more harm than
giving a tummy ache. Sugar consumption has been associated with
negative changes in cholesterol,[1] heart disease,[2] impaired learning and memory,[3] and accelerated aging. Sugar consumption in
America (and the Western world) has dramatically increased over
the last two hundred years. According to *Forbes Magazine* sugar

consumption in the United States increased from fewer than 10 pounds per person per year in 1820 to over 130 pounds per person per year in 2012.[4]

How does sugar consumption accelerate aging? There appear to be several potential pathways. At the end of chapter 4 we discussed telomeres and cellular replication. As telomeres shorten, cells lose the ability to replicate—the shorter the telomeres, the shorter the remaining lifespan. A study published in 2014 documented that individuals with high sugar consumption had shorter telomeres in their white blood cells when compared to individuals with lower sugar consumption.[5] These differences remained after controlling for sociodemographic and health-related differences. So one factor in how high sugar intake may accelerate aging is by shortening telomeres.

Another factor is that diets high in sugar typically are composed of more refined, highly processed foods. Such diets are generally lower in micronutrients, vitamins, minerals, and healthy molecules such as fiber and flavonoids. Without an ongoing supply of the building-block molecules the body needs to produce its varied different tissues, the cells fatigue, wear out, and die easier. So a second factor in how a high-sugar diet accelerates aging is by decreasing the intake of vital nutrients necessary to keep the body operating at peak efficiency.

It is well documented that long-term patterns of living (lifestyle choices) that increase inflammation will accelerate aging, reduce brain volume, and increase dementia risk. This is because chronic inflammation damages the body's tissues, including the brain, leading to the changes associated with Alzheimer's disease. We will describe the inflammatory cascade contributing to Alzheimer's disease in detail in chapter 14. And in the next section we examine one pathway in which chronic high sugar increases inflammation and accelerates aging and dementia risk. But what is less commonly known is that brief exposure to high-sugar intake also impairs memory and learning. A recent animal study found that one week of consuming a diet high in sugar impaired memory. The researchers documented that the high-sugar intake increased inflammation in the brain cells (hippocampus) where new memories are formed, thus impairing their function and causing memory deficits.[6] Therefore, reducing the consumption of sugar in the diet will both provide immediate benefit and reduce your risk of dementia in the long term.

Glycation

Another factor in how sugar accelerates aging, which has significant scientific validation, is that increased sugar in the diet results in increased oxidation via a mechanism called *glycation*. Glycation is the process of a glucose (sugar) molecule binding to other molecules such as proteins and DNA where it does not normally belong. When the sugar molecule binds inappropriately to a protein it forms a new compound, advanced glycation end-product, or AGE. AGEs react with body tissues to produce free radicals and reactive oxygen species (ROS). Both AGEs and high-sugar (sucrose) intake trigger the immune system to increase chemokines, cytokines, and other inflammatory factors (as described in chap. 5), all of which increase oxidative stress on the body. Remember, oxidation is the process of oxygen atoms binding with other molecules and damaging them. Therefore, these unnatural oxidizing molecules are damaging to our bodies, including skin, blood vessels, nerve cells, and other organs, and just as the acronym AGE suggests, they ultimately accelerate the aging process.

Here's an example. Hemoglobin is the molecule in our red blood cells that carries oxygen. But when glucose binds to hemoglobin in this unnatural way a new compound is formed called *hemoglobin-A1C* (HGB-A1C). This new aberrant molecule is highly damaging, causing injury to cells throughout the body. The higher the blood sugar levels, the higher the abnormal AGEs. Diabetics, with higher than normal glucose levels, have elevated levels of HGB-A1C with increased oxidative damage that causes many of the problems common to diabetics—neuropathy (damage to the nerves in the body that causes burning or numbness), retinal damage (causing vision problems), kidney damage, and dementia.

These inflammatory molecules also damage collagen (the protein in the body that provides elasticity, pliability, and strength). When AGEs bind to collagen in the skin they cause the skin to thin, wrinkle, and lose elasticity—accelerating aging![7]

AGEs bind with LDL (low-density lipoprotein) cholesterol, forming plaques in the walls of blood vessels, and the AGEs impair the body's ability for our good cholesterol, HDL (high-density lipoprotein), to remove the plaques. AGEs alter vascular permeability and blood flow, contributing to vascular disease and the subsequent health problems associated with vascular compromise such as heart attacks and strokes, and thereby accelerate aging.[8]

Obviously, anything that impairs blood flow to the brain would have both short- and long-term negative consequences. The blood brings oxygen, nutrients, and energy molecules to the brain and also removes waste products. A compromised circulation would undermine normal metabolism and brain function. But most significantly, impaired blood flow can result in strokes—the death of brain cells due to loss of blood to that brain region. When the blocked blood vessel is large it results in a large stroke, and most of us have seen the sad results of these—paralysis of one side of the body and often the loss of normal speech. What many people don't realize is that chronic inflammation, with subsequent plugging up of the arteries with plaques, increases the risk of not only large artery strokes but also small vessel strokes. The small vessel strokes do not cause the paralysis or sudden loss of speech but instead cause the loss of a few neurons or neuron-to-neuron connections. Over the course of years these small losses add up to big losses and cause vascular dementia—dementia due to the blood vessel disease that obstructed blood flow causing the death of neurons.

Clearly, elevated levels of advanced glycated end-products are damaging to our bodies and contribute to accelerated aging as well as the risk of dementia. So what are the sources of these AGEs and how can we reduce them?

The two primary sources of glycation are the body's own metabolism and the foods we eat. The greater our consumption of sugary foods, the greater concentration of sugar molecules in the body, which results in increased production of AGEs. Anything that increases the blood sugar levels will increase the body's production of advanced glycation end-products. Sugar-filled snacks, foods with high glycemic index, and foods containing high fructose corn syrup all increase the production of these damaging molecules.

Certain forms of cooking and food preparation will form AGEs before we even eat the food, and then our bodies will absorb about 30 percent of the AGEs that we ingest. Foods high in these damaging molecules are fried foods, charred foods, and grilled foods. Examples of such foods are fried chicken, grilled burgers, seared steaks, French fries, and caramelized onions. Eating such foods increases inflammation and thereby accelerates aging.

A simple way to reduce AGEs in your body is to reduce the consumption of sugar, high fructose corn syrup, fried foods, and charred and grilled foods. Slow cooking such as using a Crock-Pot, cooking with water, and boiling foods avoids the formation of glycated proteins from cooking. Additionally, eating complex carbohydrates and foods high in fiber reduces the production of these toxic molecules in the body.

Dietary scavengers that help clear your body of these glycated proteins include apples, broccoli, spinach, kale, collard greens, peaches, cabbage, cauliflower, tomatoes, carrots, citrus fruits, most berries, omega-3 fatty acids, rhodiola rosea, green tea, grape seed extract, carnosine, and vitamin B_6.

Many people know that sugary diets are unhealthy yet have struggled to move to a healthier, less-sugar-rich diet. This may be due to the ability of high-sugar diets to change the brain's reward circuitry such that healthy foods are not as enjoyable or pleasurable as they would have otherwise been.[9]

Imagine working in your yard one afternoon and after several hours you find yourself ravenously hungry. You are pleasantly surprised when your spouse brings you a snack of perfectly ripe fresh strawberries. Can you imagine how sweet and refreshing one would taste? But now consider if you had just finished swallowing your last bite of a candy bar and your spouse offers you the same strawberries—how would one taste now? What is the difference? Has the sweetness of the strawberries changed? No, your ability to experience the sweetness of the strawberries has been changed. By eating a candy bar, or any other food with *unnatural* sweetness (artificially concentrated levels of sugar), we overstimulate the brain's reward circuits so that foods with natural sweetness are no longer as enjoyable, pleasurable, or desirable as they would otherwise be. If we do this on a rare occasion the taste receptors reset quickly, and in a few hours we can enjoy the strawberries. But if we do this chronically we actually lose "taste" for healthy foods and develop cravings or tastes for highly toxic and overly sugary-sweet foods. Thus our diets will gravitate toward patterns of eating that will accelerate aging. If we choose to change our diets and consistently eat healthier foods we retrain our brains, and the foods we initially found distasteful will become enjoyable. This usually takes about three months.

Perhaps you know people who were diagnosed with high blood pressure and instructed to eat a low-salt diet. Initially, they may have complained that the food tasted bland, but if they stuck with the new diet, after several months of low salt not only did food taste good again but also food with the previous levels of salt typically tasted too salty. Research documents that this change in taste preference takes about three months.[10]

Another example can be found in people who switched from sugary sodas to diet sodas. Initially most find the diet sodas less enjoyable, but if they continue to drink the diet sodas over months they come to prefer them to the sugary sodas. Why? Because our taste receptors and reward pathways change based on our experience. Unfortunately, diet sodas are no healthier and, in fact, may contribute to a greater risk of dementia than the sugary ones. One large study of more than five hundred thousand people ages fifty to seventy-one followed for ten years found drinks with artificial sweeteners increased rates of depression, whereas drinks with sugar or honey did not.[11] Recent research on depression has documented that one of the underlying pathways that causes depression is increased inflammation. Thus, anything that increases inflammation will increase depression risk as well as dementia risk. This is likely the reason that having a history of depression increases the risk of dementia—both problems are being caused by chronic inflammatory cascades damaging brain tissue and interfering with normal brain function.

Soft drinks have other age-accelerating effects besides the sugar they contain. Several studies have linked soft drink consumption with accelerated bone loss, which may contribute to osteopenia and osteoporosis as we age.[12] Colas were found to be more likely to contribute to such bone loss.[13] Not surprisingly, studies have linked increasing intake of sugary soft drinks with increased obesity and type 2 diabetes—both of which accelerate aging.[14] And interestingly, even when individuals drank diet soft drinks that used artificial sweeteners rather than sugar, obesity rates still increased.[15] Why might this be? No firm conclusion exists at this point, but one possibility is that these substances also artificially stimulate the brain's taste receptors and reward circuitry and may result in natural, healthy foods being less enjoyable, thus leading to dietary choices that overall are unhealthier.

Junk foods and fast foods such as pizzas, hot dogs, doughnuts, cookies, cakes, and so on increase inflammation, promote insulin resistance, and increase the risk of diabetes and obesity. All these factors accelerate aging and increase the risk of dementia later in life. But decades before dementia occurs, these unhealthy lifestyle choices cause other problems undermining well-being. Studies show that individuals who eat junk food regularly have a 40 percent higher rate of depression than those who do not eat such foods. And the impact was dose dependent, meaning the more junk food consumed, the greater the likelihood of depression.[16] This is most likely due to the elevation in inflammation triggered by such food choices.

Diets high in sugar and trans fats (trans fats are produced industrially when hydrogen is added to vegetable oils to turn liquid oils into solid fats; they appear as "partially hydrogenated oils" on food labels) accelerate aging through multiple mechanisms: (1) glycation increasing oxidative damage to body and brain, (2) increased obesity, which further increases oxidative damage, (3) diets lower in essential nutrients, and (4) altered taste reception driving toward a more sugary diet.

What lifestyle changes can we make—besides simply reducing sugar intake and eating more whole foods—that will slow the aging process, including aging of the brain?

Fasting

Have you ever fasted? I have always wondered why they call it *fasting* when the time goes by so slowly! Regardless of how slow it seems to pass, research has documented that caloric restriction or intermittent fasting slows aging, improves brain health, and prolongs life.[17] The mechanism for this appears to be via a reduction in oxidation and inflammation.[18]

Historically, the reason our morning meal is called *breakfast*, which literally meant to "break the fast," is because there was a fast between dinner and breakfast. The easiest way to implement fasting into your life is to implement a daily twelve-hour fast between dinner and breakfast. Not only does such a regular fast appear to slow aging, but one small study also showed that a daily twelve-hour fast, in conjunction with other lifestyle changes, improved memory and cognition in individuals who had *already lost abilities*. In this study of ten individuals who had either mild cognitive impairment or early Alzheimer's dementia, nine out of the ten persons showed measurable improvements within three to six months of entering the lifestyle program.[19]

In addition to fasting twelve hours each night, this lifestyle program included the following:

- An optimized diet (with reduced sugar consumption), anti-inflammatory in nature (i.e., low in AGEs)
- Stress management—daily meditation, yoga, and the like
- Eight hours of sleep per night
- Thirty to sixty minutes of exercise four to six days per week
- Cognitive exercises
- Low blood homocysteine levels
- Serum B-12 greater than 500
- Low blood levels of markers of inflammation (C-reactive protein)
- Low HBG-A1C
- Other specific nutritional factors to promote neuronal health

Diet and the Brain

Recent brain science examined blood markers of diet and identified three distinct dietary patterns detectible in the blood of those studied. Two patterns were associated with greater brain volume and improved cognitive performance, while one dietary pattern was associated with brain-volume loss and worsening cognitive performance. The dietary patterns associated with improved brain function and volume were either the vegan diet high in B vitamins and vitamins C, D, and E (fruits, nuts, grains, veggies) or the Mediterranean diet high in omega-3 fatty acids (fish oils). The dietary pattern associated with poor brain function and volume was the typical American diet of high sugar, fast foods, and trans fats (junk food).[20]

Diets high in or supplemented with long-chain omega-3 fatty acids found primarily in oily fish (EPA/DHA) appear to protect the brain and slow loss of gray matter. After the age of seventy the human brain generally shrinks by 0.5 percent per year. A study published in 2014 in *Neurology* that followed more than eleven hundred women for eight years found that women with the highest levels of EPA and DHA in their blood at the beginning of the study had brains that were about two cubic centimeters larger overall than women with the lowest amounts of these fatty acids. Further, the hippocampi, which is where new memories are formed, were 2.7 percent larger in women whose EPA/DHA levels were twice as high as the average. This study adjusted for other factors that could influence the participant's brain size such as education, age, other health conditions, smoking, and exercise.[21]

There are multiple potential reasons that a diet high in omega-3 fatty acids (EPA/DHA) yields better brain volume, cognition, and memory. DHA in the brain concentrates in the lipid membrane and improves neuronal fluidity, signaling, synaptic plasticity (ability to make new neuron-to-neuron connections), and neurogenesis (production of new neurons) and has a significant anti-inflammatory role.[22] Additionally, recent research published in the *Journal of the Federation of American Societies for Experimental Biology* suggests that omega-3-fatty acids from fish oil improve the function of the brain's glymphatic system, which is the system the brain uses to remove waste products, including amyloid protein—a protein that has been associated with Alzheimer's disease.[23]

EPA/DHA forms of omega-3-fatty acids are primarily found in oily fish, wild salmon, mackerel, and sardines. Omega-3s from plant sources such as flax seed are the shorter-chain form ALA, which the brain cannot use. Studies demonstrate that ALA is poorly converted in the body to the longer-chain forms: 8 percent to EPA and less than 1 percent to DHA.[24] Therefore, a healthy brain requires a diet high in the vital fatty acids, which means either a diet high in oily fish or taking daily omega-3 fatty acid (EPA/DHA) supplements.

▪ LEARNING POINTS ▪

1. The foods we eat become the building material for our bodies.
2. Diets high in sugar increase inflammation and contribute to oxidative stress on the entire body, compromising brain function for multiple reasons (vascular disease, direct oxidative damage, inflammatory cascades).
3. AGEs are unnatural toxic molecules formed when glucose binds to other molecules.
4. AGEs are damaging (oxidizing) and contribute to accelerated aging and increased dementia risk.
5. AGEs are formed by frying, searing, charring, and grilling foods and within our body by high glucose levels.
6. Artificial sweeteners accelerate aging and are associated with obesity and cognitive decline.
7. Fasting reduces oxidative stress and inflammation and slows the aging process.
8. Plant-based diets high in fruits, nuts, veggies, and vitamins B, D, C, and E or Mediterranean diets high in omega-3 fish oils are healthier than the typical American diet and are associated with greater brain volume and better cognitive performance.

▪ ACTION PLAN: THINGS TO DO ▪

1. Reduce consumption of processed sugars.
2. Reduce intake of high fructose corn syrup.
3. Stabilize blood sugar levels by eating complex carbohydrates, proteins, and a high-fiber diet.
4. Exercise thirty to sixty minutes, four to six days per week.
5. Eat vegetables and fruits raw, boiled, or steamed as water prevents the production of AGEs.
6. Limit consumption of browned, caramelized, deep-fried foods.
7. Limit meat, but when used, cook it slowly and at low temperature.
8. If meat is eaten, eat organic meats.
9. Drink water and eliminate soft drinks from diet.
10. Avoid foods with artificial sweeteners.
11. Fast twelve hours between dinner and breakfast.
12. Eat wild oily fish high in omega-3 fatty acids or take omega-3 fatty acid supplements.
13. If you have type 2 diabetes work with your health-care provider to keep your glucose levels within your target range. Normal glucose levels reduce the formation of AGEs.

7

Tobacco, Illegal Substances, Alcohol, and Aging

If You Abuse It, You Lose It

The best way to detoxify is to stop putting toxic things into the body and depend upon its own mechanism.

Dr. Andrew Weil[1]

Tobacco

As we have discovered in previous chapters, oxidation is damaging to the tissues of the body; therefore, anything that increases oxidation will accelerate aging. Tobacco is well documented to increase cancer risk, heart disease, stroke, lung disease, and circulatory problems and to alter immune response. But tobacco use also produces many oxidizing molecules and impairs the body's antioxidant enzymes. Thus, tobacco use also accelerates aging.

One evidence of the accelerated aging caused by smoking tobacco was documented by Dr. Daven Doshi and colleagues, who compared the skin of identical twins—one who smoked and one who did not. The twins were fifty-two years old at the time of the examination. They had spent their first two decades of life together, lived in the same latitude, and had similar sun exposure and jobs. The examiners used a standardized six-point scale to grade the level of skin damage of each twin: 1 = mild, 2 = mild to moderate, 3 = moderate, 4 = moderate to severe, 5 = severe, and 6 = very severe. The twin who did not smoke was rated at a 2 while the smoking twin's skin was rated at a 5![2] (Pictures of these twins can be seen at http://archderm.jamanetwork.com/article.aspx?articleid=654484.)

Illegal Substances

Yes, tobacco accelerates aging, and so do all illegal substances of abuse. Methamphetamine is perhaps the quintessential example of an illegal substance that accelerates aging. Methamphetamine damages the blood-brain barrier, the tight junctions in the vasculature that prevent damaging molecules from entering the brain. This allows for increased influx into the brain of oxidizing molecules that increase oxidative damage to the brain.[3] Additionally, methamphetamine itself directly affects signaling systems in the brain, resulting in increased oxidative stress and neurotoxicity.[4] The bottom line is that such substances accelerate aging and are damaging to the brain. (As a picture is worth a thousand words, I encourage you to visit rehabs.com, type "explore" in their search engine, and then page down and click "Before and After Drugs (Meth): The Horrors of Methamphetamine" to compare the before and after pictures of individuals who have used methamphetamine. The aging effects are undeniable.)

If you are one of the millions who are struggling with some chemical addiction, I encourage you to contact your health-care provider, call a help line, speak to your clergy—do whatever is necessary to get into professional addiction treatment. Chemical addiction is a disease with devastating consequences to your brain, but there is effective treatment available. Don't wait, get the help you need today! If you don't know who to call, then call the SAMHSA (Substance Abuse and Mental Health Services Administration) Help Line. This is a free, confidential, 24-hour, 365-day-per-year treatment referral service. The number is 800-662-HELP (4357). If you need the help, GET IT—call now!

Alcohol

While tobacco and illegal substances are fairly straightforward regarding their damaging impact on human health, alcohol is a different matter. There is substantial research on alcohol and its impact on health, but much of it is contradictory. I will break down the research into what is undisputed and what is still unclear and suggest some guidelines for a healthy approach to alcohol.

What is not disputed is that any alcohol consumption during pregnancy is damaging to the developing fetus.[5] It is also undisputed that heavy alcohol consumption (2.5 beers or thirty-six grams of alcohol per day or more) is damaging to body and brain, accelerates aging, and contributes to increased risk of dementia.[6] Alcohol consumption in quantities that lead to drunkenness is oxidizing and unhealthy. And it is generally understood that alcohol consumption during childhood and adolescence interferes with normal brain development. Studies have documented differences in various brain structures in people who have used alcohol during the developmental period compared to those who have not.[7]

Where things are less clear is for those adults who are mild-to-moderate drinkers. Overall the data suggests that those who drink mild-to-moderate amounts of alcohol have lower risk of dementia and cognitive decline than either problem drinkers or total abstainers.[8] It is not fully understood why this is the case, but other research has suggested some possibilities. Problem drinkers, those who drink heavily and in whom alcohol has caused health, social, occupational, or other life impairments, and those who abstain from alcohol completely have higher rates of cognitive impairment from vascular causes (strokes and microvascular damage).[9] This suggests that mild-to-moderate alcohol consumption may reduce the risk of vascular-related dementia. Other suggested reasons for the cognitive decline in problem drinkers are the direct neurotoxic effects of heavy alcohol use, which cause changes in brain structure, and brain trauma as problem drinkers are more prone to accidents and injuries. Additionally, problem drinkers suffer from deficiencies in essential nutrients, contributing to further body and brain problems. It has been known for more than a century that thiamine (vitamin B_1) deficiency in chronic alcoholics causes a form of dementia known as Korsakoff syndrome. Deficiencies in other vital nutrients may also play a role in cognitive decline in problem drinkers.

There also appears to be a difference in health based on the type of alcohol one drinks. The most beneficial effects of mild-to-moderate alcohol consumption are experienced when drinking wine, and the most damage occurs from drinking spirits (distilled alcohols).[10] This may be due to the fact that wine, red more than white, contains many antioxidant molecules such as polyphenols and flavonoids, which are lost in distilled spirits.[11] This leads to the possibility that the health benefits found in alcohol are not from the alcohol itself but from the various antioxidant compounds found in it, and these benefits persist despite the alcohol, not because of the alcohol. This is supported by studies that demonstrate that the same health benefits are observed in alcohol-free wine.[12] Further support for the idea that the benefit to the brain may not be from the alcohol itself comes from research documenting that low-to-moderate alcohol consumption does not reduce the risk of cognitive decline. The researchers who found alcohol consumption was not associated with cognitive benefits suggest the reason some studies found what appeared to be a benefit "may have been due to inclusion of former drinkers in the abstainers reference category."[13]

Another confounding fact with alcohol use is its long-term impact compared to its immediate effect. The immediate effect of alcohol is relaxation, euphoria and sedation, impaired response time, and reduced motor control, which are experienced with either a buzz or intoxication. These effects occur because the alcohol physically interacts with the neuronal membranes, altering the functioning of the neurons in real time. As the concentration of alcohol goes up, the more neural membranes are affected and the greater the intoxicating effect. As the alcohol is cleared the physical impact on the neurons is removed, and the effects of intoxication clear. However, alcohol also activates a cascade of second messengers inside neurons that cause delayed effects. Like kicking over dominoes, these second messengers send signals down to the DNA within the neurons of the brain's alarm circuitry (amygdala), altering gene expression that causes the alarm circuit of the brain to be more reactive. In other words, during intoxication one feels more relaxed because of the immediate physical effects of the alcohol on neuronal membranes, but once the alcohol clears one can experience increased anxiety due to the alteration in gene expression in the amygdala.[14] This can be one factor that contributes to an increased craving for more alcohol.

With all these variables in mind and considering how the body is designed to prevent alcohol from reaching the brain, it really does raise the question of whether there are genuine brain-health benefits from alcohol. When we consume food and drink, it passes through the mouth, down the esophagus, into the stomach, and then into the intestines for processing and absorption into our bloodstream. The blood then transports the processed ingested substances throughout the body. But immediately after absorption into the bloodstream and before distribution throughout the body, the blood travels directly to the liver. And the liver is chock-full of various enzyme pathways designed to metabolize and render inactive a wide variety of potentially harmful substances. The body is built this way to prevent potential brain-altering toxins from ever reaching the brain and impairing functioning. In order for a substance to impact the brain it must first get past the liver. One enzyme pathway contained within the human liver breaks down alcohol into water and carbon dioxide. This is because alcohol is a by-product of some bacteria living in the gastrointestinal system.[15] The body is designed to protect the brain, to keep it highly functional and alert. When we eat carbohydrates some of them are metabolized by the bacteria in our gut, forming small amounts of alcohol. This alcohol is absorbed with the rest of the nutrients and transported to the liver, where the liver detoxifies the alcohol into water and carbon dioxide. The water is excreted in the urine and the carbon dioxide exhaled from the lungs and, when things function normally, no alcohol reaches the brain. Perhaps mild-to-moderate drinkers gain benefit from the antioxidant molecules in the wine they drink, but because of the enzymes in the liver that detoxify the alcohol, the alcohol has minimal impact upon the brain itself. But heavy drinkers bombard their bodies with frequent and damaging amounts of alcohol, causing a wide variety of health-compromising effects, including accelerated aging and cognitive decline.

Putting it all together, then, we can draw the following conclusions regarding alcohol:

- Any alcohol consumed during pregnancy is damaging to the developing fetus and should be avoided.
- Any alcohol consumed during brain development (childhood and adolescence) is damaging and should be avoided.
- Heavy alcohol use (2.5 drinks per day or more) at any age is unhealthy and should be avoided.

- If one chooses to use alcohol, mild-to-moderate wine use has the greatest evidence of benefit, but this benefit is likely due to the polyphenols and not the alcohol.
- Distilled spirits have no evidence of health benefit and have high risk of harm.

▪ LEARNING POINTS ▪

1. Tobacco in all forms damages health, increases oxidation, and accelerates aging and should be avoided.
2. Illegal substances of abuse are oxidizing and accelerate aging and should be avoided.
3. While research on alcohol is mixed, when balancing all the various risks of alcohol consumption (risks of falls, accidents, bleeding, cancer, addiction, etc.) with the potential reduced risk of cardiovascular and neurocognitive problems, and then weighing in the evidence that documents the same health benefits can be obtained by consuming nonalcoholic wine, the best health recommendation to reduce *all* the various health risks is to avoid alcohol and use nonalcoholic wine. But if one does use alcohol, mild-to-moderate amounts of wine for nonpregnant adults with no medical contraindications, history of addiction, addictions in immediate family members, or any cognitive problems would be best.

▪ ACTION PLAN: THINGS TO DO ▪

1. If a tobacco user, stop—see addendum for smoking-cessation strategy.
2. Do not use alcohol while pregnant.

3. Do not drink alcohol before age twenty-one.
4. If you use alcohol, avoid distilled spirits and limit use to no more than two drinks per day.
5. Do not use alcohol as a treatment for anxiety—if you have anxiety that needs treatment see your health-care provider.
6. If struggling with chemical addiction, whether drugs or alcohol, get help! If you don't have immediate access to help in your community, then call the SAMHSA (Substance Abuse and Mental Health Services Administration) Help Line. This is a free, confidential, 24-hour, 365-day-per-year treatment referral service. The number is 800-662-HELP (4357). If you need the help, GET IT—call now!

PART 3

LIFESTYLE
AND AGING

8

Exercise and Your Brain

If You Don't Use It, You Lose It

I get bursts of creativity with bursts of physical
activity.

Payal Kadakia[1]

want you to do an experiment. Use a stopwatch or clock with a
second hand, and for just one minute—only sixty seconds—sit
perfectly still. Not just quiet, not with minimal movement, but
don't move one muscle in your entire body (other than breathing)—don't blink, don't shift, don't turn your head, don't swallow.
Try it. What happened at the end of that one minute? Did you find
you had some urgency to move?

We are designed for movement, for activity, for exercise. Yet our
modern world has interfered with healthy exercise. Ancient humans
exercised as part of daily life. Survival required exercise—long
hunting trips, often walking or running great distances, working long hours in the fields planting and harvesting crops. Just

the routines of gathering firewood and water, washing clothes, preparing food (grinding flour, kneading bread, etc.), and even walking outside to the privy required movement. Those who didn't exercise often didn't live very long. Almost all of life's activities required significantly more exertion—exercise—than life requires today. But the benefits of exercise have been known for millennia. In China around 2500 BCE, it was noted that exercise prevented certain diseases termed "failed organs." These diseases were perhaps diabetes and heart failure. The writings of Confucius promoted exercise and various gymnastics. Martial arts with daily, regimented routines were introduced and are still practiced by large segments of the Chinese people today. The Chinese also enjoyed other physical activities such as badminton, archery, dancing, and wrestling.

In India, a form of yoga was developed that is the most commonly known form in the West and is a series of various body postures and positions requiring regular physical exertion. It was recognized in ancient India that regular exercise was necessary for optimal health.

Perhaps no ancient society has had greater impact on physical fitness in the West than ancient Greece. The Greeks not only found the human body beautiful and the object of art but also promoted the development of physical fitness. Ancient Greeks developed the Olympics, and some Greek scholars such as Hippocrates and Galen spent their lives studying the human body and promoting physical health. However, much of their influence was lost with the fall of the Roman Empire and the breakdown of organized society.

During the Dark and Middle Ages life consisted of hunting, gathering, maintaining shelter, and tending cattle. Exercise was required if one was to survive. Those not fit enough to engage in the physical rigors of life, unless they were from quite wealthy families, would typically die.

Tribal life in the Americas was similar. Exercise was required for survival. Even those who didn't hunt and gather would carry heavy loads, tan leathers, set up dwellings, cut wood, and prepare food. Life prior to the modern industrial revolution was a life of nearly constant physical exertion.

The founders of the United States recognized the importance of regular exercise. Benjamin Franklin said, "Use now and then a little Exercise a quarter of an Hour before Meals, as to swing a Weight, or swing your Arms about with a small Weight in each Hand; to leap, or the like, for that stirs the Muscles of the Breast."[2] And Thomas Jefferson is noted for recognizing the value of regular exercise, and not just for the health of the body; he also realized that a healthy body promoted a healthy mind. Following are three of his noteworthy comments:

> Exercise and application produce order in our affairs, health of body, cheerfulness of mind, and these make us precious to our friends.[3]

> Walking is the best possible exercise. Habituate yourself to walk very far.[4]

> A strong body makes the mind strong.[5]

From the founding of the United States in 1776 throughout the nineteenth century, the vast majority of life's activities required daily physical exercise. The industrial revolution, however, changed life drastically. Modern machinery reduced the amount of physical labor required for almost every task. The cotton gin, steam engines, tractors, automobiles, trains, dishwashers, washing machines, dryers, and vacuum cleaners have reduced the amount of exercise required for vast segments of society.

Indoor plumbing and electricity further reduced physical activity. Elevators reduced stair climbing; cable cars, buses, subways, and automobiles cut down on walking. Manufacturing plants and assembly lines drew people from agricultural life to city living, resulting in standing in place for long hours. And all this modern living has contributed to an epidemic of diseases never before seen in society—diabetes, hypertension, hypercholesterolemia, heart disease, and obesity—all of which accelerate aging and undermine brain health. Please don't think I am suggesting humanity was better off before the industrial revolution—not at all. I am only saying that along with many blessings to humanity, the industrial revolution also brought an unforeseen consequence—reduced physical exercise with subsequent worsening health.

The good news is we are still free to exercise. Whereas prior to the industrial revolution exercise was part of daily living, for most of us today we must choose to make exercise part of our lives. If we do, the benefits are enormous.

Benefits of Physical Exercise

Regular resistance and aerobic exercise increase muscle strength, cardiovascular fitness, and bone density.[6] And the benefits of exercise are realized at every age. The Fitness Arthritis and Seniors Trial (FAST) demonstrated that older adults who exercise are 40 percent less likely to develop disability than those who do not exercise.[7]

We not only have fewer disabilities as we age if we exercise, but we also reduce inflammation in the body. Regular aerobic exercise causes the muscles to produce the powerful anti-inflammatory factor interleukin-10.[8] This factor suppresses inflammatory cytokines known to contribute to increased risk of depression, dementia, vascular disease, diabetes, obesity, and some chronic-pain conditions.

Regular exercise causes the brain to produce at least three different neurotrophins (brain-derived neurotrophic factor, nerve growth factor, and vascular endothelial growth factor). These proteins cause the brain to make new neurons, stimulate existing neurons to sprout new connections, and provide support in maintaining the health and vitality of our brain cells.[9] Older persons who exercised regularly saw 2 percent growth in the hippocampus of their brains. This is the part of the brain in which all new learning takes place. As I mentioned previously, *this new growth reversed approximately two years of aging!*[10] Let me emphasize this last point. Exercise resulted in growth in the part of the brain in which new memories occur, and the new growth was the equivalent to turning the clock back two years! In this study participants started out walking ten minutes per day at a faster pace than their normal walking speed and increased each session by five minutes each week. At the seventh week they were walking forty minutes per day.

Animal studies reveal the same results. Active animals have larger hippocampi, which means they can learn faster than sedentary animals.[11] And older people who walk just fifteen minutes per day have a lower risk of Alzheimer's dementia.[12] People who routinely exercise exhibit better cognitive abilities and sharper memory and have larger brains than people who do not routinely exercise.[13]

Physical exercise provides all the benefits listed above, and the circuits of the brain that initiate movement (striatum) also initiate thinking. This is why persons with Parkinson's disease, which is caused by the loss of cells in the striatum, have not only slowed physical movement but also more difficulty initiating thoughts.[14] And while scientists have known for years that the cerebellum coordinates our physical movements so they are smooth, organized, and balanced, more recent research has documented that the cerebellum also coordinates our thinking.[15] This means that physical exercise not only improves brain volume but also enhances the circuits of the brain involved in initiating, organizing, and coordinating our thought processes. This is why sparks of insight often occur when people are exercising. It is also an important reason for children to get regular physical activity; as they exercise they develop the circuits of the brain that not only help motor control but also improve thinking and cognitive control.

Every organ and motor system of the body has as its primary purpose to serve the brain—to provide oxygen, nutrients, and data input to the brain or to move the brain from place to place or to carry out the desires and intentions of the brain. It is no wonder, then, that maintaining a healthy body has such a huge impact on the health of the brain.

Exercise is a requirement for life. It is a design law—a parameter on which life is constructed to operate. If you want something to get stronger, you *must* exercise it. As we discussed in chapter 2, if you want stronger muscles, you must exercise them. If you want stronger math ability, you must work problems. If you want stronger musical skill, you must practice your instrument. This is the law of exertion—strength comes from exercise. Or as it's more commonly put: *use it or lose it.*

Benefits of Mental Exercise

While it is true that we must exercise the body in order to be healthy, to have the healthiest brain possible we must also exercise our minds.

When we choose to practice a musical instrument we direct neural circuits to fire that are associated with that activity. The more we fire them, the more neurotrophins (brain-produced fertilizers for the neurons) are released in those specific circuits and the more neurons and neuron-to-neuron connections are made, thus increasing the complexity of the brain circuitry, which corresponds with increased capacity and efficiency of whatever behavior one is practicing. And sure enough, the brains of musicians have been found to be structurally different from the brains of nonmusicians in areas that correspond to fine motor activity and auditory and visual processing.[16] The brain adapts and changes as a result of our choices for every activity of life. To maintain a healthy brain we need to exercise both our bodies and our minds.

We can exercise our minds by reading new material that requires thinking and contemplation and learning new concepts. Write, do puzzles, engage in new physical activities such as art or learning to play an instrument, playing ping-pong, learning to waltz, or learning a new language. Mentally stimulating activities and certain brain-training programs are associated with lower brain amyloid levels (a protein associated with Alzheimer's) and a decreased risk for AD, as are graduating from college or engaging in lifelong learning.[17]

Physical Exercise Recommendations

See Your Doctor!

First and foremost, before starting any exercise program see your doctor, get a physical exam, and discuss your plans with your health-care provider. Starting an exercise routine after years of sedentary living can be dangerous and actually cause injury, so it is important to *start low and go slow*. This means to start with low intensity, low weights, and low repetitions and increase slowly. Overdoing it can cause muscle, bone, joint, and tendon injuries as well as potential life-threatening problems for those with serious cardiovascular disease. Therefore, step one is to *see your doctor* and together formulate a plan to get you back in top physical shape.

Choose Exercises That You Find Enjoyable

After seeing your doctor, step two is to choose exercises that you find enjoyable, not stressful.

Anecdotal reports have been around for years of individuals who exercise but who don't experience improvement in metabolic health—they don't lose weight and they don't experience improvement in lipids or glucose control. This led health-care providers to doubt their patients who reported they were exercising.

However, in 2012 a study of 1,687 individuals revealed that 10 percent of people who exercised regularly experienced worsening cardiovascular and diabetes risks.[18] This may be due to the mindset of the person doing the exercise. When we are stressed the brain activates the amygdala (stress circuit), which in turn activates the hypothalamic-pituitary-adrenal axis, increasing stress hormones. The stress hormones activate the immune system, increasing chemokines, cytokines, and other inflammatory factors. It is well documented that chronic activation of this inflammatory cascade contributes to worsening cardiovascular and metabolic risks, including worsening diabetes and obesity. Therefore, one potential reason that a subset of people who exercise regularly do not experience benefit is that they may be exercising with a mind that is stressed; they may dread or dislike the exercise and thereby worsen the inflammation in their body.

A very simple fix is to choose physical activities that you enjoy. Make the exercise a by-product of the activity, such as playing tennis, racquetball, walking while golfing, hiking, dancing, or rowing while fishing. Another way to make exercise more enjoyable is to make it a part of a group experience—walk together with family or friends or join an exercise class. If none of these work for you, consider exercising while listening to audio books that you look forward to hearing. Doing these things shifts the mind's focus away from the exercise and onto the game, the friends, the beauty of nature, or the story, which in turn changes the emotional experience from one of stress and dread to one of fun and joy.

Be Balanced!

While it is well documented that too little physical activity undermines health, recent research has demonstrated that too vigorous exercise also undermines health, increasing oxidative stress. Those who engage in extreme exercise routines such as marathon running, iron-man competitions, and the like have the same mortality rates as those who don't exercise at all.[19]

Recommendations for optimal exercise include:

- Moderate aerobic exercise five days per week, thirty minutes per day (ten-minute bouts), or vigorous aerobic exercise three days per week, twenty minutes per day
  - On a scale of 0 (sitting) to 10 (all out), moderate = 5, vigorous = 7–8
- Strength training at least two days per week
  - Eight to ten different exercises; at least one set of ten to twelve reps each
- Flexibility two days per week, ten minutes per day[20]

▪ LEARNING POINTS ▪

1. If you don't use it, you lose it—the law of exertion; if you want something to be stronger, you must exercise it.
2. Regular physical exercise reduces inflammation and causes the production of multiple proteins that promote brain health, reducing the risk of dementia and other disabilities.
3. Brain circuits that initiate and organize physical movement are the same circuits that initiate and organize our cognitive abilities.
4. Regular mental exercise keeps the circuits of the brain active and healthy and reduces the risk of dementia.

▪ ACTION PLAN: THINGS TO DO ▪

1. See your doctor, get a physical exam, and discuss with your doctor your exercise plan.

2. Choose exercises that are sustainable and enjoyable.

3. Ensure some aerobic activity (walking is sufficient) a minimum of fifteen minutes per day.

4. Get an exercise partner or join an exercise group—the encouragement of friends can keep us going on those days we are not as motivated.

5. Engage in lifelong learning—stimulate your mind to contemplate new ideas, learn new skills, or develop new abilities.

9

Sleep and Your Brain

A Requirement for Life

> Early to bed, early to rise makes a man healthy,
> wealthy, and wise.
>
> attributed to Benjamin Franklin

The corollary of exercise is the need for rest. In this chapter we will explore the importance of physical rest—sleep, what normal sleep is and is not, the amount of sleep people need at different ages, and the health consequences when people don't experience routine restorative sleep. In the next chapter we will examine the incredible benefits of regular mental rest (rest for the mind) on our physical, mental, and brain health. Both types of rest are essential for good health, and failure to regularly experience sleep and mental rest accelerates aging and increases the risk of dementia.

So let's start with physical rest—sleep. There are four physical requirements to life—air (I bet you knew that one), water, food, and sleep. The first three everyone instinctively knows, but it is surprising how many people don't realize sleep is a physical requirement for life and health. Alterations in normal sleep always have negative health consequences—it is unavoidable.

According to the Centers for Disease Control (CDC) in Atlanta, sleep deprivation in America is becoming epidemic. Over forty-nine million Americans report sleep difficulties that impair concentration, more than eighteen million report memory problems related to sleep loss, and over forty million Americans report impairments in daily functioning related to such things as work, hobbies, finances, or driving.[1] People with chronic sleep problems suffer higher rates of diabetes mellitus, obesity, hypertension, depression, and cancer and die younger than those who get normal sleep (which we will discuss shortly).[2] The CDC's analysis of the prevalence of sleep problems found that 34 percent of people sleep fewer than seven hours per night, 48 percent report snoring, 37.9 percent report unintentionally falling asleep during the day, and 4.7 percent report falling asleep while driving.[3] The US Department of Transportation estimates there are 100,000 accidents, 1,550 fatalities, and more than 40,000 injuries each year due to drivers impaired by sleepiness.[4]

While we are awake our brain cells are very active. Even though the brain weighs only about three pounds, which is 1–2 percent of the body weight, it uses 20 percent of the body's energy. This high metabolic activity means the brain is producing by-products of metabolism that need to be removed from the brain. The waste removal occurs during sleep. When we are asleep our brain cells contract, expelling the by-products of metabolism from the fluid (cytoplasm) inside the neurons out into the cerebrospinal fluid to be removed from the brain.[5] If we don't get normal amounts of sleep we interfere with the brain's ability to remove these metabolites. Over time this can contribute to increased oxidative stress and neuronal loss, accelerating the aging process.

This is why infants, toddlers, children, and adolescents need more sleep than adults—their brains are assimilating more data and structurally going through much more modification and change. Thus, they have more by-products of metabolism to clear.

According to the National Sleep Foundation, recommendations for sleep by age are as follows:[6]

Newborns (0–3 months)	14–17 hours
Infants (4–11 months)	12–15 hours
Toddlers (1–2 years)	11–14 hours
Preschoolers (3–5 years)	10–13 hours
School-age (6–13 years)	9–11 hours
Teenagers (14–17 years)	8–10 hours
Young adults (18–25 years)	7–9 hours
Adults (> 25 years)	7–8 hours

Unfortunately, many people don't get normal amounts of sleep, and this not only impacts physical health but also undermines mental health, accelerates aging, and interferes with learning. According to data from the National Health Interview Survey, nearly 30 percent of adults reported an average of fewer than or equal to six hours of sleep per day in 2005–7.[7] And according to the CDC, in 2009 only 31 percent of high school teens reported getting at least eight hours of sleep on school nights.[8] And sleep deprivation not only impacts health but also undermines learning. A study by Dr. Kyla Wahlstrom at the University of Minnesota demonstrated that pushing school start times back from 7:15 a.m. to 8:40 a.m., which allowed for increased sleep time, resulted in less depression, better attendance, and less tardiness.[9] Further, improved sleep resulted in fewer auto accidents, less obesity, and better grades.

Additional studies have confirmed the role sleep plays in memory consolidation and learning. Nicolas Dumay published research in the journal *Cortex* in 2016 that demonstrates marked improvement in declarative memory and recall when periods of learning were followed by sleep. In two studies participants were asked to memorize made-up words. Then they were asked to recall those words immediately after exposure and twelve hours later. Those who slept during the intervening twelve hours were not only able to recall more words than those who didn't sleep but also able to recall more words than they did immediately after learning them twelve hours previously.[10]

But it is not merely the number of hours slept during each twenty-four-hour day that is important. Studies also show that *when* one sleeps is critical to optimum health. Sleeping at night, in harmony with nature's biorhythms—awake when the sun is up and asleep when the sun is down—is much healthier than working during the night and sleeping during the day. In fact, according to research that followed almost seventy-five thousand registered nurses over twenty-two years, those who worked third shift for five years or more died younger and had significantly higher rates of heart disease than those who did not work third shift; and those who worked third shift for fifteen years or more died at higher rates from lung cancer than those who worked the day shift.[11] So not only is sleep a physical requirement for life and health, but also *when* one sleeps is critical to maintaining optimum health and to slowing the aging process.

What Is Normal Sleep?

Now that we have examined the amount of time a person needs to sleep, let's explore what normal sleep is. There are four basic stages to sleep. When a person first falls asleep they enter stage one sleep. This is a very light sleep when people often don't even think they are yet asleep. This is when Grandma is snoring on the couch and the grandchildren say, "Grammy, you're snoring!" Grandma startles and says, "What? No I wasn't; I wasn't even asleep." Many people in stage one experience sudden muscle jerks called *hypnic myoclonia*, often associated with a sensation of being startled. Stage one sleep is relatively short, and if not awakened in stage one a person quickly enters stage two sleep.

In stage two sleep eye movements stop and brain waves slow down, and there are characteristic brain-wave spikes that can be seen on an electroencephalogram (EEG) called *sleep spindles*. Stage three sleep is the deeply restorative slow-wave sleep (previously divided into stages three and four sleep but now considered one stage) in which the body temperature falls and heart rate slows. A person in this stage is difficult to awaken. There is no eye movement or voluntary muscle activity (other than the diaphragm for breathing) during this stage of sleep. If awakened during this stage people are often initially confused and disoriented. I remember a somewhat embarrassing experience I had because of being awakened during this stage of sleep while I was in my residency.

I did my residency in the US Army at Eisenhower Army Medical Center at Fort Gordon, Georgia. As active-duty army soldiers, my fellow residents and I had to not only provide routine patient care but also maintain military readiness in case of deployment. Therefore, we had periodic readiness alerts in which, at random and unpredictable times, the alert roster was activated. These alerts often seemed to happen in the middle of the night. I was a lowly captain, home obliviously asleep, when one night my telephone rang and startled me awake. I am certain I must have been in stage three sleep because I was confused and disoriented and have vague memories of answering the phone when my commanding officer identified himself. But I simply could not register the meaning of what he was saying. I kept repeating very loudly and apparently rudely to the colonel, "Who are you? Who are you? Who are you?" This went on for a minute or so before I realized to whom I was speaking and then began apologizing profusely. Fortunately for me, my commander was a psychiatrist who understood sleep stages, and while I was not in any trouble, it made for quite a funny story the next morning.

It is in stage three sleep that some individuals experience bed-wetting, night terrors, and sleepwalking. During stage three the body is working to build muscles and repair damage that occurred from work and exercise. Thus, if one has had a particularly hard workout or engaged in extra physical labor, their sleep may be a little deeper that night.

Stage three is followed by REM (rapid eye movement) sleep. REM sleep is the stage in which dreaming occurs. During REM sleep the brain cuts off signals to the body's muscles so that a person doesn't physically act out all the various activities they are dreaming about. This normal lack of movement during dream sleep is lost in up to 80 percent of cases of both Lewy body dementia and Parkinson's disease, causing REM movement sleep disorder. [12] This sleep disorder can precede the onset of Parkinson's or Lewy body dementia by a decade or more. Those with AD, rather than having movement problems during REM sleep, have decreased and fragmented periods of REM sleep.[13]

During normal REM sleep our eyes move rapidly, body temperature rises back to normal, and breathing increases. REM sleep is when memories are consolidated. During the day when we learn new information this retention occurs in the part of the brain called the *hippocampus*. During sleep information is transferred from the hippocampus to other cortical regions for long-term storage. The complete relationship between memory and sleep is not fully understood. But it does appear that REM sleep is critical to consolidating memories with significant emotional content.[14] It is also during REM sleep that significant emotional issues are processed by our sleeping minds. Such emotional energy contributes to the content and quality of our dreams. But what happens when REM sleep ends (and this is critical to understanding what normal sleep is)? When REM sleep ends—we wake up! When REM sleep ends we do not immediately go back into stage one sleep, but instead there is a brief awakening. Then after this awakening we enter stage one sleep and start another REM cycle, which ends with another brief awakening.

From the time a person enters stage one until they awaken at the end of REM is anywhere from 70 to 120 minutes. These wake-ups between REM and stage one are normal, and everyone experiences them. When we are young or extremely sleep deprived or physically exhausted, these wake-ups may last only a few seconds as we shift or turn and then fall right back to sleep. Often we have no memory of waking up, and therefore we falsely believe we slept all night. This leads people to think that healthy sleep is when we sleep seven to eight hours solid with no awakenings. But as we age and these normal awakenings occur, we often get the clarion bladder call and have to make a trip to the bathroom. Because we remember these wake-ups we begin to worry we are not getting good sleep. This can lead people to start using medications they do not need and which can actually worsen sleep architecture and sleep quality and contribute to memory and cognitive problems.

I have many patients present to my office complaining of not sleeping well, when their only change is remembering these normal wake-ups. Their problem is not abnormal sleep but the worry and heightened anxiety they now have because they *think* they are not sleeping well. Once I educate them on normal sleep and their mindset shifts, things improve. Most adults need five of these cycles per night, which results in seven to eight hours of sleep per night. If you get five of these cycles per night—even if you have multiple wake-ups—as long as the wake-ups are natural and occur between REM and stage one, then your sleep is normal and no treatment is necessary.

Human Sleep before Electricity

There is one other aspect to normal sleep patterns that has recently been discovered. Prior to electricity and modern illumination, the sleep pattern for much of humanity was not one solid eight-hour period of sleep. Rather, historians have documented that, especially during winter months with long nights and shorter days, sleep naturally occurred in two four-hour bouts with a one-to-three-hour interval of wakefulness in the middle of the night.

Walter Brown, MD, clinical professor of psychiatry at Brown University, correlating historical data uncovered by A. Roger Ekirch, professor of history at Virginia Polytechnic Institute, has documented that natural sleep patterns throughout much of human history were quite different from what modern societies experience. Prior to electricity and artificial lights, sleep typically occurred in two separate bouts, known as first sleep and second sleep. Each period consisted of about four hours and was anchored to sunset and sunrise. People would typically go to bed shortly after sunset, sleep for about four hours, arise for one to three hours, then go back to bed around 1:00 to 2:00 a.m. and arise near sunrise. During the middle of the night people engaged in a variety of activities—reading, writing, socializing, household chores, and so on. This two-bout pattern of sleep has also been observed in animals such as apes and giraffes and was recently confirmed to still occur in certain primitive tribal communities in Africa where artificial illumination is not available.[15]

The importance of recognizing this is that normal sleep is not a solid block of uninterrupted sleep but rather consists of five to six REM cycles punctuated by awakenings between each and may be experienced in two separate blocks each night.

Sleep and Medicines

Failure to recognize the normal sleep pattern has resulted in many patients and health-care providers seeking to medicate normal sleep patterns to artificially instill a solid block of supposedly uninterrupted sleep. However, this is not only frequently unnecessary but may very well be harmful and contribute to more cognitive and memory problems.

Many of the common medicines used to promote sleep have known risks of increasing cognitive and memory problems and the risk of dementia. Common prescription sleep medicines are in the family known as benzodiazepines. These include antianxiety medicines such as alprazolam (Xanax), diazepam (Valium), clonazepam (Klonopin), and lorazepam (Ativan), as well as sleep agents (sedative hypnotics) such as triazolam (Halcion), flurazepam (Dalmane), temazepam (Restoril), zolpidem (Ambien), eszopiclone (Lunesta), and zaleplon (Sonata). There have been eleven studies looking at the risk of benzodiazepine use and dementia. Nine of these studies have shown a positive risk, one study showed no risk, and one study showed reduced risk.[16]

The preponderance of the evidence at this time would suggest that these sleep medicines increase the risk of dementia. This is likely due to chemical signaling interference of memory transfer during sleep. During learning all new information is stored in the hippocampus of the brain. During sleep this information is transferred from the hippocampus into the cortex for long-term storage. Two possible mechanisms may be contributing to the increased memory and cognitive problems from benzodiazepine use during sleep. First, these medications may chemically interfere with neural signaling and may mechanically prevent the neural activation necessary for memory consolidation.[17] Second, benzodiazepines alter normal sleep architecture, increasing the amount of time in stage two sleep while reducing the time in stage three and REM sleep.[18] Therefore, using benzodiazepines nightly for sleep increases the risk for cognitive and memory problems immediately while simultaneously increasing the risk for dementia later in life.

Another class of medications used for sleep and often available over the counter are antihistamines such as diphenhydramine (Benadryl). One of the brain's primary wake-promoting chemicals is histamine, produced in the brain stem and released into the prefrontal cortex. Thus, antihistamines produce sleepiness in most people. The problem with most antihistamine medications, however, is that they are not pure antihistamine. Instead, they have many other actions, and it is these other actions that contribute to most of the memory and cognitive problems associated with these medicines. For instance, diphenhydramine and hydroxyzine (Vistaril) are not only antihistaminic but also highly anticholinergic, which means they block receptors in our brains and bodies that respond to the neurochemical acetylcholine. Acetylcholine is important in memory and learning. In fact, the brain's primary center for acetylcholine production (mammillary bodies) is damaged in Alzheimer's dementia, and medicines used for Alzheimer's dementia that are designed to help improve memory such as donepezil (Aricept) work by increasing the availability of acetylcholine. So chronic use of antihistamines that also have strong anticholinergic effects contributes to memory and cognitive problems. And these impairments are worse the older a person is.

It is unknown how many people may have normal sleep—with middle awakenings—but believe they are not sleeping well and therefore seek either over-the-counter sleep aids or prescription sedatives, which actually contribute to cognitive and memory problems and increase the risk of dementia. If you are currently taking medicines to promote sleep consider speaking with your doctor to reevaluate the need for such medicines.

One of the most common nonmedical substances used to assist with sleep is alcohol. While alcohol, the proverbial nightcap, can result in faster sleep initiation, it reduces the amount of time in stage three and REM sleep, which often results in early awakenings and interferes with memory consolidation. Therefore, alcohol as a sleep aid is not an option for those seeking to be the healthiest they can be in order to reduce cognitive and memory problems.

Sleep Apnea

Of the many sleep disorders, one deserves discussion here—obstructive sleep apnea (OSA). OSA is a disorder in which, during sleep, the muscles in the throat relax and the soft tissues obstruct the windpipe (trachea). The diaphragm tries to pull in air, but the windpipe is obstructed and no air enters the lungs. The oxygen level in the body falls, and when it reaches a certain point an alarm fires in the brain stem that awakens the person who tightens the muscles in the throat. A breath is taken, the oxygen level increases, the alarm turns off, and the person falls back asleep. However, this process results in the person oscillating in and out of the early stages of sleep and not progressing through the deep restorative and REM sleep phases. This interferes with the body's normal circadian release of various body hormones, energy production, memory consolidation, glucose metabolism, and fat metabolism.

Untreated sleep apnea increases the risk of hypertension (high blood pressure), heart disease, type 2 diabetes, obesity, asthma, reflux, and car accidents.[19] Additionally, OSA is associated with increased risk of depression, loss of gray matter in the brain, and cognitive and memory impairments.[20] The good news is that re-search shows that treatment of OSA, typically with a face mask connected to a machine that increases the air pressure in the airway and thus prevents the soft tissues from closing the windpipe, known as a CPAP (constant positive airway pressure), results in reversal of the loss of brain tissue and memory and cognitive problems.

Sleep Assessment and Simple Interventions

When evaluating a person who is struggling with achieving normal sleep it is important to assess any factors that could be promoting wakefulness or interfering with sleep. Common factors include the following:

- Room temperature—typically people sleep better in a cool room.
- External noises—are there environmental noises that inter-fere with sleep? If so consider a sound machine or ear plugs.

- Physical health problems such as pain conditions, frequent urination, breathing problems, infections, itching—optimizing treatment for any such condition is essential for maximizing sleep efficiency.

- Animals in the room—I am astounded at the number of my patients who complain of sleep problems, yet when I take their history they readily endorse having a pet that routinely wakes them up. Amazingly, many of them, rather than make changes in their homes to limit the animal's ability to wake them (i.e., keep the pet out of the bedroom), instead seek medications to sedate themselves so that they won't be awakened.

- Caffeine—caffeine has an average half-life of six hours (reports range from three to nine hours),[21] which means it takes six hours to clear 50 percent of the current level of caffeine out of the body. So if at 6:00 a.m. a person consumes 200 mg of caffeine, there will be 100 mg in their body at noon, 50 mg at 6:00 p.m., 25 mg at midnight, and 12.5 mg at 6:00 a.m. the next morning. Caffeine does not give a person energy but instead blocks the receptors that register the brain signal that one is tired, fatigued, and in need of sleep. Thus, for individuals who have sleep problems it is important to remove caffeine.

- Nicotine—nicotine before bedtime can cause increasing alertness and interfere with sleep; many persons who are nicotine dependent enter nicotine withdrawal about four to six hours into sleep, which can cause awakening in the middle of the sleep period.

- Irregular sleep schedule—establishing routine go-to-sleep and wake-up times helps train the brain and body to sleep. And the most crucial anchor point is the wake-up time. The adult brain wants to be awake sixteen hours per day, so if one sleeps in until 10:00 a.m. the brain won't want to go to sleep until around 2:00 a.m.

A recent study documented the benefits of regular exercise on improving sleep time and quality, even when the exercise was in the evening hours. The study found that evening exercise was associated with improved objective sleep and more deep sleep, shortened sleep-onset time, and fewer awakenings.[22] If you struggle to get normal, restorative sleep, take a careful inventory of your daily routines, identify potential factors that may be interfering with sleep, and then make interventions to resolve those factors. If sleep problems persist, talk to your physician.

▪ LEARNING POINTS ▪

1. Sleep is a physical requirement for life.
2. The amount of sleep required changes with age.
3. Normal sleep includes periodic awakenings that do not require medicating.
4. Adults need seven to eight hours of sleep per night.
5. Many sleep medications worsen sleep quality, interfere with memory and cognition, and may contribute to dementia.

▪ ACTION PLAN: THINGS TO DO ▪

1. If you have sleep problems do a sleep inventory and eliminate factors known to interfere with sleep. If problems persist see your physician.
2. If you feel chronically fatigued, have frequent headaches or memory or cognitive problems, are known to snore, or wake up excessively, then speak to your doctor about the need for a sleep study to evaluate possible sleep disorders.

3. Review your medication list with your doctor and discuss changing meds known to contribute to thinking or memory problems or that interfere with normal sleep architecture.

4. Do not use alcohol or sleep products that contain alcohol for sleep as alcohol interferes with normal sleep and contributes to memory problems.

5. Engage in routine exercise that not only promotes brain health but also improves sleep quality.

6. If you have sleep problems remove known stimulating agents from your diet (such as caffeine) even if you slept well for years drinking the same level of caffeine. As we age our body metabolism changes; doses of caffeine we could metabolize and clear when young may contribute to sleep difficulty when older.

10

A Vacation in Time

Rest for the Mind = Health for the Brain

Time is the coin of your life. You spend it. Do not allow others to spend it for you.

Carl Sandburg, at his eighty-fifth birthday party, January 6, 1963

Richard didn't want to come see me. He was by all accounts a high-functioning, successful executive for a Fortune 500 business. His entire life he had succeeded in whatever he put his mind to. He had an MBA, graduating with honors, and was able to secure a job with a desirable company after graduation. He worked long hours and produced outstanding results and over his career was rewarded with bonuses, promotions, and advancements. Yet, in his fifties he was in my office and was not happy to be there.

A typical day for Richard went like this:

- 5:00 a.m. awaken, shower, shave, dress
- 5:15 coffee and pastry, review emails, check the news
- 5:45 out the door, drive to work
- 6:15 arrive at office, begin workday (business lunch or no lunch)
- 6:00 p.m. leave office, drive home (stop to do errands when needed)
- 6:30–7:00 arrive home
- 7:00–9:00 microwave meal, yard work, address problems with wife that presented during day (home repairs, family issues)
- 9:00–10:30 work on computer related to office job
- 10:30–11:30 watch TV, often news
- 11:30–12:00 a.m. go to bed

Weekends were not much better. While he would sleep in a couple of hours longer, he would spend much of his time working on his computer or doing chores around the house. Very little time was spent in simple relaxation and mental rest, allowing himself to unwind and lay aside the burdens of life. Even when he went to church on Sundays (he didn't go every week), he had his smart device with him and would read or do business on his device while there.

Richard's life is typical of how many Westerners live: overworked and little time for simple relaxation and rest—not sleep for the body, but rest for the mind.

In my practice the vast majority of my patients identify themselves as practicing Christians. Yet most of these individuals do not get regular rest. Those who attend church typically set aside the burdens of living only for a few hours on Sunday mornings. As soon as church is over, they go right back to the grind. My patients almost always tell me they would like to have a day off each week just to relax and rest, but they cannot afford it—there is simply too much to do. Working five days a week and having kids in school who are engaged in numerous extracurricular activities, they feel obligated to use their day of worship for catching up on shopping, housecleaning, laundry, and yard work. They feel like rats in a wheel—a wheel that never ends and running a race with no finish line.

Do you ever feel this way?

Research has documented that overwork, working long hours without adequate time for mental rest, increases physical and mental health problems. A meta-analysis of over six hundred thousand adults found that overwork is associated with increased risk for heart attacks and strokes.[1] Death due to work-related stress has become so common in Japan that their culture even has a name for it—Karoshi. This problem had become so pervasive in Japan and disability claims had become so common that in 2002 the Japanese government released guidelines on limiting work hours.[2] Not only does overwork and failure to get proper mental rest contribute to heart attacks and strokes but also such persistent mental stress alters DNA expression and increases cancer risk. A study that examined the impact on DNA of work-related stress and perceived overwork found, particularly in women, that these resulted in increased damage to DNA, increasing the risk of cancer.[3]

Maintaining One's Health

I see many good-hearted people who have burned themselves out because they simply don't know how to say no—how to set boundaries, how to take time to rest.

One of the traps that caring people fall into is doing too much. Many of my Christian patients get tricked into exhaustion because they fear being selfish or that any action they take to care for themselves before others will be viewed as selfishness. So they never say no but instead take on more and more until they are burned out.

Such individuals have failed to understand how reality works. This is the law of rest-oration. When a finite being expends a resource, that being must rest and recover in order to assimilate more of the resource to expend again. After pitching a no-hitter a major league pitcher must rest before he is ready to pitch another game. After expending mental and emotional energy we must rest and rejuvenate before we are ready to expend more; to do otherwise leads to exhaustion. We cannot care for anyone else if we ourselves are incapacitated. Parents can only give to their children when they are in a position to give. If a parent is in an ICU on a ventilator they are not able to give to their children. If a pastor wants to nurture his congregation he must be in a healthy enough state to do so. Thus, the first principle in all altruistic activity is to maintain the health of the giver.

Even Christ took time away from the masses for rest, rejuvenation, and time in meditation and conversation with his Father. Healthy self-care is not selfish but necessary in order to keep oneself in the best condition for the maximum benefit and usefulness one can provide—in whatever activity one chooses to engage.

By understanding this principle we can gain some insight into why the Bible prescribes a weekly Sabbath rest—a weekly twenty-four-hour period to lay aside the burdens and stresses of life and rest. This rest is not the physiological sleep our bodies need each day but the rest our minds need to unwind, decompress, and rejuvenate. This type of rest is like a weekly vacation in time (a sabbatical), a day each week when a person can set aside their burdens, work, and responsibilities and rest without guilt, without feeling lazy, and without a sense of shirking one's duties because one realizes this is time—like sleep for the body—that is necessary to maintain one's own health and wellness. This time of rest for the mind, this period of rejuvenation can be a time filled with activities that further recharge and repair the body and mind.

Such activities include spending time with family. Studies show that individuals with close family ties have lower stress levels, solve problems better, and have overall better health and fewer mental health problems than individuals with fractured and strained family relations.

And science documents that vacations with spiritual emphasis are physiologically healing and slow the aging process. A recent study of 102 women ages thirty to sixty found that a five-day vacation with meditation improved stress regulation, immune function, and telomerase activity (which lengthens telomeres and slows aging) and had other positive cellular changes. These changes were immediate, and for those who continued meditation the benefits continued ten months later. The vacation and meditation turned down inflammation and calmed the immune system.[4]

When people leave their home and go away the change in environment allows them to relax, let their defensive posture down, and reduce their stress response, all of which impact genetic expression and cellular function. One can enjoy a weekly Sabbath rest at home by engaging in walks in nature, visitation with family and friends, and worship of God. Prepare the home before the beginning of the rest period by cleaning and organizing, removing and reducing stressful life cues (TV and electronic media are turned off, schoolwork is put away, etc.), and bringing out environmental cues that signal calm and rest (candles, special foods with heartwarming aromas, music reserved for the day of mental rest, etc.). Such a weekly vacation in time can promote profound health benefits.

Weekly Rest and Aging

Dan Buettner traveled the world seeking out the places where people lived the longest, the places with the highest concentration of individuals living over one hundred years of age. He termed these areas blue zones and authored the bestselling book *The Blue Zones*. He identified lessons from all the blue zones that contribute to longevity and health. The only blue zone in the United States is Loma Linda, California, which is home to a high concentration of Seventh-day Adventists. One of the lessons noted on the Blue Zones website that contributes to longevity among the Adventists is a weekly Sabbath rest. The Blue Zones website states:

> Find a sanctuary in time to decompress. . . . Observance of the Sabbath strictly occurs from Friday to Saturday night, giving Adventists a weekly time to focus on family, friends, God and nature.[5]

The weekly day of rest provides multiple health benefits. It is a time to not only mentally decompress but also get out into nature, visit with family and friends, and spend time in spiritual development. All of which slow aging and lengthen life.

Nature and the Body

Recent scientific research has documented significant health benefits to getting out into nature. Spending time in more natural, less urban environments has been demonstrated to reduce stress, improve mood, lower aggression, decrease hostility, and overall improve both mental and physical health. A study of 498 Japanese individuals evaluated the impact of walking in the forest versus a routine day. The study found hostility and depression scores decreased significantly, and liveliness scores increased significantly on the forest day compared with the control day.[6]

Further research found that when Japanese men spent three days and two nights in a forest, not only did their subjective emotional sense of well-being improve but also their heart rate variability improved, and their bodies experienced a shift in neurological stress tone. Their parasympathetic activity (which governs rest) increased and their sympathetic activity (which governs the stress response) decreased. Additionally, their stress hormone levels (salivary cortisol) and heart rates decreased markedly while in the forest setting.[7] A study of over eleven thousand Danes confirmed the association between time spent in nature and improved physical and mental health.[8]

Research has demonstrated not only the health benefits of spending time in outdoor natural settings but also that such settings seem to improve learning. In Great Britain over one hundred schools have been established that operate in outdoor forest settings. Observation of students from these schools noted improvements in the children's confidence, motivation and concentration, language and communication, and physical skills.[9]

Noise Pollution

There are multiple reasons why time relaxing in nature is more beneficial than time in more urban settings. One of the reasons is that urban centers are noisy, and noise greater than 65 dB has been associated with a host of health-related problems. Our brains are wired to alert us to potential dangers. When you hear a loud bang you startle before you even think about what just happened. The brain is wired so that loud sounds directly activate its fear/stress circuitry to alert us to potential danger. While this is helpful in natural settings where loud sounds are rare, in urban settings where noise is constant this automated pathway results in ongoing chronic activation of our brain's stress circuitry, even if we are not consciously fearful or stressed.[10] Thus, chronic noise exposure does result in increased stress activation with subsequent increased inflammation and increased rates of heart attacks and early deaths.[11] A study that examined the impact of traffic noise on preschoolers (ages three to seven) found that children who attended preschool in zones with high traffic noise (>60 dB) had higher mean systolic and diastolic blood pressure than children in quiet areas.[12] And a study evaluating the impact of aircraft noise on learning found that chronic aircraft-noise exposure was associated with higher levels of noise annoyance and poorer reading comprehension measured by standardized scales.[13] Thus not only is health impacted by noise (>60 dB) but learning is also impaired.

The Balance of Electrons

Another factor in why getting back to nature may promote health is the electrical modulation that nature has on the human body and brain. Doctors have known for many years that the human organism has not only biological processes (DNA, RNA, proteins) but also electrical ones. When a doctor administers an ECG (electrocardiogram) he is recording the electrical signal patterns of the patient's heart. An EEG (electroencephalogram) is a measure of the electrical activity of the brain. Our bodies are bioelectric machines and as such are subject to electrical forces. The human brain responds to external electrical signals. One of the most effective treatments for major depression is electroconvulsive therapy; more recently strong electric magnets have been demonstrated to be effective for treating depression in persons who have not found success using multiple antidepressant medications.[14]

Our bodies suffer when imbalances in natural design occur, whether they are nutritional (scurvy caused by lack of vitamin C), hormonal (hypothyroidism—too low thyroid hormone), circadian (jet lag or night-shift work), or, as recent research suggests, electrical.

Since the middle of the twentieth century, due to the mass production and use of electrical-obstructing materials (rubber, plastic, etc.) and modern living conditions, vast numbers of humans in Western societies have essentially been unplugged from the earth. The earth is a massive bioelectric sphere that constantly gives off electrons, most spectacularly seen in blazing bolts of lightning. When human beings come into direct contact with the earth— walking barefoot in the grass, swimming in the ocean, touching a tree—the individual is "grounded" and electrical balance is achieved. Research has demonstrated that coming into direct contact with the earth with one's skin results in immediate changes in the electrical condition of the human body and restores a healthy natural balance. This process has come to be called *earthing.* Earthing has been shown to generate immediate changes in EEGs, surface electromyography (SEMG), and somatosensory evoked potentials (SSEPs).[15] But this contact needs to be with electrically conductive materials such as moist soil, grass, trees, and plants and not most man-made surfaces such as sidewalks, asphalt, and rubber-containing playground surfaces.

Research has demonstrated that daily contact with the earth provides the body with electrons that help the body establish and maintain its normal circadian rhythms and activates the body's anti-inflammatory and antioxidant enzymes, thereby reducing free radicals and damaging reactive oxygen species (ROS).[16] It is thought that the influx of electrons into the body by routine contact with the earth results in reduction and elimination of damaging oxidative chemicals.[17] Earthing results in measurable improvements in immune response, reduction in cytokines and other inflammatory markers, and improvement in recovery after injury or heavy exertion.[18] Contact with the earth also results in measurable improvements in blood flow throughout the body, with subsequent improvement in oxygenation.[19] Other studies have demonstrated that earthing or "grounding" people so that they experience this daily electrical reset results in improvement in sleep, reduction in pain, normalization of cortisol levels, less fatigue, better energy, lower blood pressure, and reductions in stress as measured by EEGs, electromyograms, and blood-volume pulse.[20]

Not only does spending time in nature seem to provide multiple health benefits but also exercise conducted outdoors rather than indoors appears to have a more robust health benefit. A twin study revealed that when physical activity was conducted outdoors it resulted in significantly lower rates of depression than when exercise occurred indoors.[21] A multistudy meta-analysis of over twelve hundred individuals found that outdoor exercise resulted in substantial improvement in self-esteem and mood.[22] And multiple studies have demonstrated beneficial differences in physical responses such as heart rate, blood pressure, autonomic response, and endocrine markers from outdoor exercise.[23]

At least one study has documented that improved autonomic response can be achieved with indoor exercise *if one views scenes of nature* while exercising.[24] This demonstrates the significant impact our thoughts, minds, beliefs, and mental attitudes have on our physiology. (In the next chapter we will explore the impact our beliefs have on physical and mental health and the aging process.)

Cheerfulness Is Good Medicine

As we discussed in chapter 8, it is not just the specific activity that matters but the mental attitude one has during the activity that is of utmost importance. Exercise with a negative mental attitude can actually cause increased stress cascades and worsen rather than improve health.

Likewise, it is not sufficient to merely avoid work one day in seven to experience health benefits; one must do so with a positive mental attitude. Weekly rest performed from a sense of obligation—under some sense of religious requirement in which the mental attitude is one of restriction, coercion, or force—damages instead of rejuvenates. Mental attitudes that incite fear and anxiety cheat people from experiencing the benefits that a weekly rest would otherwise provide. Imagine you go on vacation but in your mind you believe you are being imprisoned against your will. No matter the location, such a mental construct will incite fear and anxiety and damage your health, not improve it. So too if persons belong to religious groups that make their day of rest obligatory, a restriction of liberty, a day in which behaviors are monitored with fear of condemnation. Rather than experiencing a health benefit, their health is potentially damaged.

This is why the Bible teaches that genuine benefit from Sabbath observance occurs only for those who experience the day as a delight (Isa. 58:13–14)! And recent science confirms the ancient wisdom of Solomon that a cheerful attitude is good medicine, but a negative attitude undermines wellness (Prov. 17:22).

Researchers have found that those who laugh regularly have significantly reduced risk of heart attacks. In fact, cardiologists at the University of Maryland found that patients hospitalized with heart attacks had a history of being 40 percent less likely to laugh than persons not suffering heart attacks.[25] Laughter has been documented to improve vascular function and release of nitric oxide, which helps dilate blood vessels and improve blood flow. Conversely, mental stress, worry, and anxiety degrade nitric oxide and contribute to vascular constriction and reduced blood flow. Laughter improved blood flow by 20 percent whereas stress decreased blood flow by 35 percent.[26] Other research found that in individuals who had suffered a heart attack, humor reduced recurrence. In fact, those in the humor group had fewer arrhythmias, lower blood pressure, lower urinary and plasma stress hormone levels, less use of nitroglycerin for angina, and a markedly lower incidence of recurrent heart attacks when compared to those not in the humor group.[27] Additionally, regular laughter has been documented to improve the body's immune system and reduce the risk of infections.[28] Yes, our mental attitude really does matter!

▪ LEARNING POINTS ▪

1. Unremitting mental stress contributes to burnout and increased inflammation in the body, which increases oxidation and accelerates aging—including aging of the brain.

2. The law of restoration requires finite beings, after the expenditure of energy, to rest and recover. Violation of this law results in exhaustion, burnout, and even early death.

3. A weekly vacation in time in which one puts aside the stresses of day-to-day living and decompresses reduces inflammation and is associated with longer life.

4. Healthy activities include constructive time with family and friends, meditation and worship, and time in natural settings.

5. Regular physical contact with the earth has positive health benefits through electrical grounding of the body.

6. Engaging in health-promoting activities from a sense of obligation incites stress and undermines health.

▪ ACTION PLAN: THINGS TO DO ▪

1. Set healthy limits for work and job responsibilities at sustainable levels to prevent burnout.

2. Take a weekly vacation in time to rest your mind.

3. Spend regular time in natural settings, appreciating the beauty of nature.

4. Touch the earth, walk on the beach or grass, put your hands on the stalks of plants, swim in the ocean, river, or lake.

5. Be sure to engage in all health-promoting activities from a sense of freedom, cheerfully celebrating with family, friends, and God; avoid a rules-oriented approach that incites anxiety and stress.

6. Arrange to do your daily exercise outdoors, in a natural setting, then stretch and cool down with bare feet on the grass or beach or by wading in water.

7. And laugh, find the humor in life, take time to smile, and develop a cheerful attitude.

11

Our Beliefs and Aging

The Healthiest Worldview

We can have no surer sign of the decay of a
province than to see Divine worship held therein
in contempt.

Niccolò Machiavelli, *Discourses on Livy*, 1517

One of the principles that has made America great is freedom of conscience—that each person has the fundamental right to choose their own beliefs and that it is a violation of human rights to coerce others into believing or observing religious practices. As reasonable and logical as this sounds to our modern minds, when the Constitution of the United States and the Bill of Rights were written such ideas were truly revolutionary. Throughout most cultures in human history coercive pressure was brought to bear upon people to force conformity to the culturally accepted religious norm.

Just a cursory review of human history is filled with the abuse, torture, and execution of people based on a difference of religious belief:

- Old Testament Israel stoning people for blasphemy
- Babylonian King Nebuchadnezzar ordering people to bow to a golden idol or be burned to death in a fiery furnace
- Jewish persecution of followers of Christ
- Roman persecution of Christians
- Crusades in which Christians warred against Muslims
- The Inquisition
- Catholic persecution and execution of Protestants
- Protestant persecution and execution of Catholics
- The Puritans, intolerant of limited reforms in England, fleeing religious conflict and landing at Plymouth Rock
- The Salem witch trials at which Christians from a mainly Puritan background burned at the stake women accused of witchcraft
- American Christians persecuting Mormons
- Hindu and Muslim conflict in Pakistan and India
- Jewish and Islamic wars
- Persecution of Jews throughout history
- Persecution and execution of Buddhist nuns and priests in China during the ninth century CE[1]
- Islamic extremism in the world today

Truly, the institutionalization of religious freedom into the very foundation of American law was an absolutely radical yet genius concept. This single principle of liberty, of freedom to think and choose for oneself, is one of the core concepts that has contributed to the rise of the United States as one of the greatest nations in history.

The principle of liberty is an essential reality to how God designed human beings to function, and the New Testament overtly teaches that when it comes to religious beliefs, "each . . . should be fully convinced in their own mind" (Rom. 14:5). However, it is a mistake to confuse the fact that people have the freedom to choose their beliefs with the false idea that all beliefs are equally healthy. They are not! Some beliefs are positively harmful.

Not All Beliefs Are Healthy

Believing cigarette smoking improves health and that tobacco is beneficial as a medicine and helps one breathe better, something doctors thought for years,[2] is not as healthy as believing cigarette smoking damages the lungs and contributes to a wide variety of diseases.

History is replete with accounts of people who acted with sincerity and a genuine interest to help but who believed something unhealthy and therefore, regardless of intent, injured rather than healed. For more than two millennia physicians practiced bleeding and leaching to drain "evil humors," wrongly believing sickness was due to some mysterious bad substance in the blood. George Washington, after falling ill, had half his body's blood drained, certainly accelerating his demise.[3]

In the nineteenth century doctors used a variety of poisons such as quinine, arsenic, calomel (mercury), antimony, and strychnine to treat a broad range of conditions.[4] They called these toxins "medicines." But believing these poisons promote wellness is not as healthy as realizing they kill!

And if treating patients over the years with "purging, puking, poisoning, puncturing, cutting, cupping, blistering, bleeding, leeching, heating, freezing, sweating, and shocking"[5] were not bad enough, psychiatry jumped in with the infamous lobotomy early in the twentieth century to treat a variety of mental, behavioral, and emotional problems.

False beliefs that result in injury are not restricted to medicine. On October 30, 1938, panic broke out across North America as millions believed the world was being invaded by martians. Orson Welles's dramatization of *War of the Worlds*, broadcast nationwide on CBS radio, was thought to be real, and "civilians jammed highways seeking to escape the alien marauders. People begged police for gas masks to save them from the toxic gas and asked electric companies to turn off the power so that the Martians wouldn't see their lights. One woman ran into an Indianapolis church where evening services were being held and yelled, 'New York has been destroyed! It's the end of the world! Go home and prepare to die!'"[6]

In 1633 the Roman Catholic Church tried Galileo and found him guilty of heresy for teaching the earth rotates around the sun. Why did the church fail to embrace the truth? Because its philosophers refused to examine the evidence. Galileo, writing to astronomer Johannes Kepler in 1610, said:

> My dear Kepler, I wish that we might laugh at the remarkable stupidity of the common herd. What do you have to say about the principal philosophers of this academy who are filled with the stubbornness of an asp and do not want to look at either the planets, the moon or the telescope, even though I have freely and deliberately offered them the opportunity a thousand times? Truly, just as the asp stops its ears, so do these philosophers shut their eyes to the light of truth.[7]

Galileo was imprisoned and kept under house arrest until his death in 1642.

Religion and Unhealthy Beliefs

History documents that religious people throughout the world have engaged in destructive practices based on various beliefs that were damaging rather than healing. Sadly this continues in a variety of ways today.

In April 2016 *The Guardian* reported on an offshoot religious sect in Canyon County, Idaho, known as the Followers of Christ, who believe that medical illnesses should be treated only with prayer and such things as rancid olive oil and wine. Brian Hoyt was a member who, as a twelve-year-old, broke bones in his foot while wrestling. His family treated him with prayer, rubbing rancid olive oil on his leg and having him drink kosher wine. He left the church after watching an infant die from an untreated respiratory infection. In 2015 NBC reported:

> Herbert and Catherine Schaible prayed and prayed, but their 2-year-old son Kent died of pneumonia in Philadelphia [in] 2009. It was bacterial pneumonia, and antibiotics could have saved him. They were convicted of child endangerment and involuntary manslaughter and placed on probation but horribly, the same thing happened again just four years later. In 2013, their 8-month-old son Brandon died, again of bacterial pneumonia.
>
> "We believe in divine healing, that Jesus shed blood for our healing and that he died on the cross to break the devil's power," Herbert Schaible said in a 2013 police statement. Medicine, he said, "is against our religious beliefs."
>
> This time the Schaibles were charged with third-degree murder, pleaded no contest and were jailed. Their remaining children went into foster care.[8]

According to a task force set up by the governor, the child mortality rate for the Followers of Christ is ten times higher than for the rest of the state.[9]

Several years ago I attended a seminar at Harvard University that focused on inclusion of spirituality in medical care. There were speakers from a variety of religious traditions—Protestant Christian, Roman Catholic, Buddhist, Muslim, Jewish, but also Christian Science. The speaker for the Christian Science tradition reported that while they will seek professional medical treatment for things such as eyeglasses, hearing aids, and setting broken bones, prayer is preferred to medicine to treat most illnesses. I went to the microphone and asked a few questions.

"If your child had bacterial meningitis would your approach be to give antibiotics and pray or to pray only?" The speaker replied that they would pray and give cool compresses and other nonmedical interventions to try to reduce the fever and keep the child hydrated and comfortable but not give antibiotics.

I then asked, "If your child was playing in the backyard and stumbled across a hornets' nest and was being attacked by the hornets and you had easy access to hornet/wasp spray, would you use the spray or would you drop to your knees and pray to God to deliver your child?" The speaker with absolute certainty in her voice immediately replied that she would use the spray. To which I replied, "Then can you explain the difference as to why you would use a man-made chemical to save your child from attack by bugs in the hornet scenario but refuse to use man-made chemicals to save your child from attack by bugs in the bacterial meningitis scenario, other than the size of the bugs?" She stood there speechless; she looked to the moderator for help and then simply shrugged and said, "I don't know."

Destructive religious beliefs are not restricted to physical illness. Today, millions of religious people live in fear, insecurity, and anxiety due to some belief they have about God.

Yes, we are all free to determine our beliefs, but freedom to choose one's beliefs doesn't determine the reliability, health, value, and truthfulness of said beliefs. Genuinely healthy beliefs are those grounded in reality, in fact, in truth, in wisdom, and in harmony with how God actually designed reality to function.

In my book *The God-Shaped Brain: How Changing Your View of God Transforms Your Life*, I documented the impact various religious views have on our brain. I will not reproduce that work here but summarize with this: God-concepts that promote love, forgiveness, compassion, beneficence, reasoning, thinking, and the pursuit of truth and evidence while respecting the freedom of conscience are healing to the brain. God-concepts that incite fear; promote hostility, intolerance, conflict, and resentment; shut down thinking; undermine reasoning; minimize truth and evidence; and lead to the coercion of others are damaging to the brain. Our belief systems really do matter. Beliefs that are grounded in reality—how life actually works and functions—and that move people toward love, forgiveness, and so on are healthiest.

The good news is that regardless of what beliefs one holds we are free to change them. We can, with examination of evidence, reason things through from cause to effect, make careful experiment, test our ideas against reality, and replace erroneous ideas for ever-increasingly more accurate ones. When we do, a positive physical transformation occurs in our brains and bodies. But clinging to unhealthy beliefs activates the brain's stress circuitry and the immune response, increasing inflammation and causing a subsequent increased risk of type 2 diabetes, heart attacks, strokes, loss of bone density, and depression, all of which accelerate aging and increase the risk of dementia.[10]

People don't like to be wrong, so unless a person has reached a certain level of maturity, a level at which they can say, "I am finite; there is an infinite universe of information (or an infinite God) and knowledge that I don't know. Therefore, while this is what I currently believe to be true, I am open to update and change my beliefs when the evidence persuades me that a new understanding is healthier, more reliable, and sustained by how reality actually functions," then their fear of being wrong not only closes their minds to healthier understandings but also often results in hostility toward others who believe differently.

This means the healthiest mindset is one that loves to grow and advance in truth as it is understood and comprehended rather than maintaining a mindset that believes it already possesses the truth and therefore resists any new insights. Those who love and seek truth are less anxious and less fearful because they are open to modifying their thinking as new credible evidence is presented. However, those who rest on tradition, custom, or established institutional constructs often experience more fear and anxiety through life from the stress of new ideas and perspectives that threaten their current view. This is especially true if they have already rejected truth in order to defend their historical stance. I have seen both scientist and theologian manifest both types of thinking—open and interested and growing in greater truth, and closed and hostile and unwilling to consider ideas that don't comport with their previously stated perspectives. What I did not explore in my previous book is the impact belief systems without God—agnostic and atheistic—have on our ability to move toward an ever-increasing reality-based understanding of the world and method of living.

Science and Unhealthy Beliefs

All human beings, whether religious or secular, scientist or layperson, can believe falsehoods and are vulnerable to being resistant to advancing truth, evidence, and new ideas. Our challenge is to develop the ability to think, reason, weigh evidence, and come to conclusions for ourselves so that we can eliminate distortions from our thinking and refine our belief systems to be more consistent with how reality functions.

Unfortunately, history demonstrates that it is not an easy thing to change beliefs. For the majority of people, once they have formed a belief, acted on that belief, and taught that belief, they become resistant to evidence that would replace the false belief with a more accurate one—even among those of science who claim their beliefs are based on observable evidence.

Scientists are also human and their minds build belief systems that can be just as resistant to new evidence that would refute their current paradigms as a pastor, priest, or theology professor would, and history proves this to be true.

In 1867 Joseph Lister, an English surgeon, after reading a paper on germ theory by Louis Pasteur, pioneered antiseptic techniques for surgery. He published six articles that year in the *Lancet* describing the new techniques: using a dilute solution of carbolic acid in sterilizing instruments, preparing the skin before surgery, washing hands before wound probing, and so on. His protocols resulted in marked reductions in postoperative infections and improved survivals. He visited the United States in 1868 and again in 1876, presenting his findings in lectures to leading American doctors. And how did US doctors respond to this evidence? They refused to believe it, which resulted in tragedy.

On July 2, 1881, James Garfield, the twentieth president of the United States, was shot by Charles Guiteau. Over the course of the next several months the top doctors in America repeatedly probed the wound track with unwashed fingers and unsterilized instruments, refusing to believe the evidence of Pasteur and Lister. Sadly, President Garfield died September 19, 1881—not from damage caused by the bullet but after a long, arduous course with infection. He was only forty-nine years of age.

Today hypertension (high blood pressure) is called the silent killer and is recognized as a serious health problem, contributing to strokes, heart attacks, renal failure, and early death if not treated. However, when high blood pressure was first discovered doctors refused to believe it was something to be concerned about.

> The greatest danger to a man with high blood pressure lies in its discovery, because then some fool is certain to try and reduce it.
>
> J. H. Hay, 1931[11]

> Hypertension may be an important compensatory mechanism which should not be tampered with, even were it certain that we could control it.
>
> Paul Dudley White, 1937[12]

Perhaps one of the greatest false beliefs scientists continue to cling to today is an idea that has its origin in ancient Greek paganism: spontaneous generation—that life originates spontaneously from nonliving matter. Even though science has proven this does not occur,[13] even though there has never been one example of nonliving matter spontaneously giving rise to life, many scientists still cling to the false belief that life began in this way. They now call it *abiogenesis* and have added a long explanation of how it might have happened, but after cutting through all the distractions the bottom line is the same: life originating in nonliving matter.[14]

For life to happen three divergent elements are necessary, and they must work together harmoniously: matter, energy, and information (organized data). Consider as an analogy a computer: for a computer to be operational there needs to be hardware (matter), electricity (energy), and software (information). The computer will not function with only two of these three elements. Nor will it work if they do not work harmoniously and in proper balance— too much energy and the circuits fry; matter that doesn't conduct energy to the proper parts or insulate in the proper places and the computer malfunctions.

All living organisms require the same. There must be matter, an energy source, and organized operational information that contains the base programming directing the functions of the operating systems of the organism. The atoms that make up the various molecules (DNA, proteins, etc.) would be the matter, energy would be from the various chemical and ionic reactions going on within the organism, and the information is found encoded within specific sequences in the DNA strands.

Scientists who deny God focus entirely upon the physical components that are the building blocks of living organisms, the DNA, proteins, and so on. They ignore entirely the complex information stored within the DNA itself. Where did that information originate? The idea that living beings originated on their own without any intelligent input would be similar to believing the following scenario: a storm arose with high winds, rain, and lightning that raged for years; during this storm the strong winds blew rocks and sand at high speeds until some were shattered and worn down and formed letters of the alphabet. This is analogous to believing that the random forces of nature mixed together in some chemical soup with lightning strikes and eventually formed DNA molecules. Even if we were to accept that this happened (which is a big leap of blind, evidence-less faith), scientists still ignore the most critical aspect of what is required for life—the encoded information contained within the organized DNA sequences. Having an alphabet does not mean we have usable and functional information. To believe that random forces brought life about would require we not only believe the alphabet formed on its own but, beyond this, that we also believe the winds, rains, and lightning strikes—all on their own—organized the letters into the entire Encyclopedia Britannica. Yet this is exactly what millions of good-hearted, honest, thinking people do believe.

But why would thinking, honest-of-heart scientists choose to believe something that the evidence refutes? Because the historical alternative belief system is significantly more destructive! What is the historical alternative belief system—the one that reasonable people reject? The belief in an all-powerful god who functions no differently than the worst despots in human history—a god who says, "Love me or I will burn you in hell forever."

This grotesque god-construct, rightly rejected by reasonable people, is pointedly described by Richard Dawkins in his book *The God Delusion*:

> The God of the Old Testament is arguably the most unpleasant character in all fiction: jealous and proud of it; a petty, unjust, unforgiving control-freak; a vindictive, bloodthirsty ethnic cleanser; a misogynistic, homophobic, racist, infanticidal, genocidal, filicidal, pestilential, megalomaniacal, sadomasochistic, capriciously malevolent bully.[15]

145

Sadly, this warped god-construct—intolerant, dictatorial, capricious, arbitrary, and severe—became the view promulgated in theory and practice by Christianity through much of history. This distorted view of God led to the complete reversal of Jesus's teaching to "love your enemies and pray for those who persecute you" (Matt. 5:44) and resulted in the Crusades, the Inquisition, burning dissenters at the stake, and the closing of millions of minds to the pursuit of truth that resulted in the Dark Ages. And the Dark Ages was a period of superstitious beliefs, irrational religious practices, and incalculable cruelty in the name of God.

The Unhealthiest Belief about God

The New Testament church lived quite differently than Christians in the Dark Ages. New Testament Christians refused to war against Rome, lived communally and in peace with their neighbors, shared to help others, and often died as martyrs. By all accounts a New Testament Christian would have made a great neighbor—helpful and kind but never pushy or judgmental, seeking to uplift but always respectful of the individuality of others. But all this changed with the acceptance of a single false idea—that God's laws function no differently than human laws, which are imposed rules that require the rule giver to inflict punishment for rule breaking.

But by recognizing God's laws as design protocols on which reality is constructed—the laws of physics, gravity, thermodynamics, health, and so on—we realize deviations from them are inherently damaging and result in pain, suffering, and death. In such a worldview God is never the source of inflicted pain, suffering, and death but is instead the Designer who seeks to heal and restore any of his creatures who will let him.[16]

In her book *Finding Truth*, Nancy Pearcey describes the problem for those who deny that nature's laws were specifically *designed* by a higher intelligence:

The origin of the universe has given rise to a puzzle known as the fine-tuning problem. The fundamental physical constants of the universe are exquisitely balanced, as though on a knife's edge, to sustain life. Things like the force of gravity, the strong nuclear force, the weak nuclear force, the electromagnetic force, the ratio of the mass of the proton and the electron, and many other factors have just the right value needed to make life possible. If any of these critical numbers were changed even slightly, the universe could not sustain any form of life. For example, if the strength of gravity were smaller or larger than its current value by only one part in 10^{60} (1 followed by 60 zeroes), the universe would be uninhabitable.[17]

These various laws are the laws the Creator put in place when he constructed and built reality. Violations of these laws are inherently destructive to those who break them—whether they believe in God or not. In day-to-day life we might simply call them the laws of health. Pearcey goes on to say: "What makes the fine-tuning problem so puzzling is that there is no *physical* cause to explain it. 'Nothing in all of physics explains why its fundamental principles should conform themselves so precisely to life's requirement,' says astronomer George Greenstein."[18] Yet millions of good-hearted, thinking people prefer to deny this reality and believe it all happened by random chance—why? Because the alternative historic view is one of an arbitrary deity whose laws are not the protocols reality functions on but are merely imposed rules enforced by inflicted punishment.

I submit that the single greatest distortion of reality in human history, the single greatest false belief that has resulted in more harm to humanity than any other, is the idea that God's laws function like human laws—which has resulted in people worshiping gods who function no differently than they do! I further submit, if Christianity had always taught that God's laws are the design parameters on which life is constructed to operate, then Christianity would not have devolved into a tyrannical, authoritarian system intolerant of diverse ideas but would have embraced the principles of liberty of conscience and encouraged reasoning and thinking, and the split with science would never have happened. There is a design law (how things actually work) in psychiatry called *modeling*, or *by beholding we are changed* (2 Cor. 3:18). This is a testable law, a design parameter on how life actually works. Our brains do rewire based on what we spend time reading, watching, thinking about, and worshiping and the activities in which we engage. If you worship a cruel, tyrannical dictator and believe it is a lack of faith to think and ask questions, such beliefs and actions will transform you into a person who is less tolerant, less open to evidence, and more willing to use force to coerce others.

This dictator version of God dominated the world during the Dark and Middle Ages and led religious authorities to resist evidence and persecute those such as Galileo who presented ideas contrary to the orthodox view.

Scientists who reject a dictator god who is the source of pain, suffering, and death have not rejected the Creator God that Jesus came to reveal but have rejected the lie, the false god that should rightly be rejected by all thinking people. The door remains open for all reasonable people, scientist or theologian, to integrate evidence, to come together and share our best ideas, insights, and evidences and then test them, eliminating those that are proven false, holding to ideas that are proven true, and keeping our minds open to possibilities not yet considered.

Why do this? Because beliefs without evidence, beliefs that are contradictory, beliefs that are not rational are damaging. There are two grand beliefs: a godless universe and a God-created universe. Under the God-created-universe theme there are two grand beliefs: a benevolent God of love and gods that are something other than love. The healthiest belief system—which results in greater health, longer life, and reduced dementia risk—is the belief in a benevolent God. The next healthiest view is a humanistic godless view in which human altruism, honesty, and freedom of conscience are valued. The worst or unhealthiest belief system is the belief in a punishing dictator god.

Our beliefs, attitudes, and thought processes really do matter; they play a critical role in our overall physical and mental health. Unhealthy beliefs increase stress and activate inflammatory pathways in our bodies and thereby accelerate the aging process and increase the risk of dementia. A study of five thousand individuals found that neuroticism—which included feelings of guilt, anger, anxiety, and depression—was associated with a greater risk for dementia. In contrast, conscientiousness was shown to be protective against dementia.[19]

Our mindset, what we think and believe, really does make a difference. Ellen Langer, a professor of psychology at Harvard, in her book *Counterclockwise: Mindful Health and the Power of Possibility*, describes her remarkable experiment that seemed to turn the clock back on aging. In 1979 she recruited men age seventy-five and placed them in a retreat in which for one week they were to pretend it was 1959—twenty years earlier. During that week they were secluded at a facility built to authentic 1959 details. They could only access reading materials, magazines, and other media that were available in 1959. And they were given IDs with their fifty-five-year-old pictures on them and instructed to pretend it was 1959. They underwent testing of physical strength, posture, perception, vision, cognition, and memory before and after this one-week retreat—and the results? In every measure they improved! They had greater flexibility, better posture, improved hand strength, improved eyesight by 10 percent, improved memory by 10 percent, and more than half even had higher IQ scores. And amazingly, when before and after pictures were shown to random strangers asking them to pick which picture the person was younger in, the strangers chose the after pictures as looking younger![20] What we think and what we think about has a real, measurable effect on our bodies and health—either improving or worsening them.

Unhealthy belief systems activate the brain's fear circuitry, which in turn activate inflammatory pathways in the body, which accelerate aging and increase the risk of dementia. This is due to chronic increased stress on our brains and bodies.

Not only does negative thinking activate stress pathways, which increase inflammation and contribute to more disease and increased risk of death, but also positive thinking has been linked to reduced risk of death. Researchers examined prospective data from over seventy thousand women and found those with the highest levels of optimism had significantly reduced risk of dying from all causes over the next eight years when compared to those with the lowest levels of optimism. The reduced risk of dying remained after accounting for variables such as healthy living practices, baseline health, and rates of depression.[21] A healthy, positive mental attitude is good for us and helps slow the aging process!

▪ LEARNING POINTS ▪

1. Respecting the freedom of conscience is a fundamental principle of mature people and societies.

2. The freedom to choose one's beliefs does not mean all beliefs are equally healthy—they are not. Some beliefs are actually harmful.

3. What we believe impacts our physical, mental, and brain health.

4. Healthy beliefs are those in harmony with how reality works (design laws).

5. Scientists and religionists are human, and both are vulnerable to believing falsehoods.

6. The unhealthiest religious belief is belief in a god whose law and government function like human law—imposed rules with inflicted punishments.

7. We become like the god we admire and worship—even if that god is not religious in nature (in psychiatry this is called *modeling*).

▪ ACTION PLAN: THINGS TO DO ▪

1. Think for yourself; don't let others form your beliefs for you.
2. Become a lover of truth, fact, and evidence with a mind open to changing your beliefs when new credible evidence is presented.
3. Pursue belief systems that promote love, compassion, forgiveness, reason, evidence, and freedom of conscience.
4. Develop the ability to love those who see the world differently than you do.

12

Mental Stress and Aging

Calm the Mind—Slow the Decline

Stressful events are inevitable, but staying
stressed is optional.

Timothy R. Jennings

Why have we heard so much about stress, reducing stress,
and stress-management techniques? Because our mental
attitudes really do make a profound impact on
our overall health and therefore can accelerate or slow the aging
process. So what is mental stress? What are some of the common
causes of it, and how can we manage it?

When we speak of mental stress we are speaking of pathological
stress such as chronic worry, guilt, and relationship conflicts that
keep our body's fight-or-flight system active. But not all stress is
harmful—in fact, some stress is healthy and necessary for growth.
When children learn to walk they are "stressing" their developing
muscles, bones, and joints. When we study any new subject we

are stressing our cognitive and memory circuits, placing demands on them, and exercising them, which results in growth and development. Healthy stretching of our abilities—healthy stress—is necessary for growth and development. It is this type of stress that leads to new insights, growth, and innovation.

It has been said that necessity is the mother of invention. Finding ourselves in need and not having an easy solution available to us increases our stress at that moment. But for the mature, such stress motivates thinking and activates imagination, problem-solving circuits, and creativity, leading to new solutions that bring innovation and development and turn off the stress circuitry. This type of situational stress is not harmful because it is self-limited, is grounded in reality, and leads to objective actions that result in growth.

The mental stress that is harmful is the stress that significantly and chronically activates the brain's alarm circuitry and sends the body into an ongoing survival state, a fight-or-flight state, often when no real, objective threat exists.

When we chronically activate the brain's fear circuitry, the brain activates our body's immune system. This happens because the immune system is to our body what our national guard is to our nation—its purpose is to protect us from invasion.

If while walking in a national park you confront a bear on the trail, your internal alarm will fire and immediately send a signal to your immune system to prepare for invasion. This happens because if you have to fight the bear to survive, you will certainly have bites and scratches with microscopic enemy invaders—germs—trying to get in. Thus, in fight-or-flight mode your body gears up your immune system to be prepared just in case microbial invasion occurs. Your immune system does this by releasing inflammatory factors such as cytokines (IL-1, TNF-alpha, etc.), which will defend you against microscopic invaders.

Under *chronic* stress the immune system stays geared up, but with no enemy invaders to attack, the inflammatory cytokines instead damage the body. Specifically, they damage insulin receptors contributing to insulin resistance. At the same time, the stress circuits of the brain are telling your body to dump more glucose into your bloodstream because you are still in fight-or-flight mode. The combined effect increases the risk of type 2 diabetes, obesity, high cholesterol, heart attacks, and strokes. All these increase inflammatory factors in the body—for example, advanced glycation end-products interfere with the body's antioxidant enzymes and thereby accelerate aging and increase the risk of dementia.[1]

Any belief system that chronically activates the fear circuitry is therefore harmful and will contribute to increased risk for dementia later in life. This includes religious beliefs that cause adherents to live in chronic guilt and fear, but it also includes secular beliefs that fail to provide relief from worry and fear of future outcomes, such as chronic anxiety about situations beyond one's direct ability to control and existential concerns such as the fear of death.

Let's examine the three major contributors to pathological mental stress and identify simple choices a person can make to lower their stress level, calm the brain's fear circuitry, lower the inflammatory cascade, and experience a healthier brain and body.

Chronic Worry

In my experience treating thousands of patients over more than two decades, the worry with which the vast majority of people struggle is the worry about controlling something that is not theirs to control. My patients never come in worrying about whether they will brush their teeth or go to work or prepare a meal for their children or shower or mow the lawn. The true duties and responsibilities that are theirs to fulfill seldom weigh them down with worry. Instead, they worry about those things in life over which they have no control—how life will turn out and what others will think about them: Will my children grow up to be healthy and responsible adults? Will I get that job? Will my house sell? Will my spouse leave me? Will he or she like me? Did they think I sounded stupid?

Studies confirm that pessimistic attitudes about future events cause negative physical changes in our bodies that undermine health and increase the chances of early death. Investigators found that those who had pessimistic and worrisome thoughts about the future had increased markers of inflammation in their blood (IL-6) and shorter telomeres (see chap. 4).[2] Both of these factors would accelerate aging and health-related problems.

Amazingly, other research has found that people who have positive mental attitudes toward aging, who are optimistic and don't live in fear of the future, live 7.5 years longer than those with more negative mental attitudes.[3] Yes, our mindsets do make a real difference in the aging process.

People worry because they forget that their true responsibility is for the decisions they make in governance of themselves, not for how things will turn out or what others will think or feel about their decisions.

Sometimes my patients worry about making mistakes, about getting "it" wrong, and this worry frequently paralyzes them into inaction. But their real fear, most often hidden from themselves, is not of making an error but of what others will think of them when the mistake is made. The true fear is fear of rejection—either in their human relationships (worrying about what others will think, afraid of offending others or being thought poorly of if mistakes are made) or in their relationship with God (worrying about what he will think, afraid of being bad or sinful or deserving of punishment if mistakes are made). Such individuals often look to others to tell them what to do so that if something turns out wrong they won't feel responsible—"He said to do it that way."

I have to educate my patients that there is a huge difference between making mistakes and choosing evil. Having a check bounce because one made a math error in their check registry is quite different from purposely writing fraudulent checks. While no mature person wants to choose evil, making mistakes is actually a healthy part of learning and growth. Life is a series of problems to be solved, and there is no evil in honest grappling with life's problems, making decisions, and then learning from one's mistakes. In fact, it is one of the primary ways we grow and develop. If a person cannot differentiate making mistakes from choosing evil they will often become paralyzed in life. Such individuals, rather than making a decision and sometimes getting it wrong and learning from the experience, will instead feel guilt, shame, and fear of rejection and will seek to avoid these negative emotions in the future—primarily by not making choices in which mistakes could be made. This causes stagnation in maturing and chronic anxiety and stress, which accelerate aging. In fact, this is neuroticism, which has been linked to increased risk of dementia as cited earlier.

Sometimes negative thought patterns are so deeply ingrained that professional help is needed to identify and change them. Consider the language you speak—how did you learn to speak? By hearing it from your environment. Your language is not biologically programmed into your DNA but was learned after birth. When was the last time you awoke and said, "Today, I am going to think in English" (if English is your primary language)? Never, it is always on and everything gets filtered through it. Our language is not the only thing we learned in this way. Many people have automated thought patterns that they learned from their childhood environment. They never choose to turn them on but they are always active, and all life gets filtered through them. Changing these automated thought patterns is similar to learning a new language; it takes purposeful effort and often someone outside yourself to teach you a new way of thinking (internal language or self-talk).

So how do we cope with the unknown future, the fear of how things will turn out, and the fear of what others will think of us? We do it by realizing we have control only over the choices we make in governance of ourselves and therefore focusing our energy on choosing to do what we believe is the healthiest, most reasonable, and most appropriate choice given the information we have at the time in any given situation. Then—and here are the three big keys to reducing stress—we (1) surrender outcomes to our higher power; (2) evaluate the results and learn from the experience by incorporating the new data into future decision-making; and (3) set other people free to think or feel any way they want about us, accept others' responses as evidence of their character, and make decisions based on that evidence on how we will interact with them in the future.

Surrendering outcomes to a higher power brings peace only if the higher power is worthy of our trust. If the God concept one holds is of a deity from whom we need to be protected (perhaps by offering him sacrifices—even offering the sinless blood of his son), then it is impossible to trust the future to such a being. If we do pray to such a being asking for their will to be done, we unavoidably live in fear because our trust has been placed in a being who is untrustworthy. Integral to resolving fear about the unknown future is reevaluating the beliefs one has about God and conforming them to qualities and characteristics that are absolutely true and trustworthy.

In our human relationships we find that we can trust people who we know from experience love us more than they love themselves and who would do anything to protect us, even give their life for us if necessary. I believe this is one of the primary purposes that Jesus Christ came to accomplish—to demonstrate such love in order to win our trust.

Unresolved Guilt

Unresolved guilt triggers the activation of the brain's fear circuitry, causing a person to stay on edge, remain hypervigilant, experience self-recriminating ruminations, and anticipate punishment or reprisal. This mental state is quite damaging and activates chronic stress pathways with subsequent activation of the immune system, increasing damaging cytokines and other oxidizing molecules and accelerating aging.

There are two types of guilt—appropriate and inappropriate. Appropriate guilt is experienced when we actually do something objectively wrong—for example, exploit another, betray a trust, and so on. Resolution of appropriate guilt occurs by learning from one's wrong choice, experiencing a change of heart attitude so you have healthier motives (this is known as repentance), forgiving one's self, making better choices in the future, and when possible and without causing further harm, seeking forgiveness from the one offended and restoring whatever damage one's actions may have caused them.

Inappropriate guilt occurs from believing a lie and is resolved by an application of the truth. A simple example of false guilt is the guilt one feels after the death of a loved one, which is often accompanied by thoughts such as "It's my fault. If I had come home earlier I could have called an ambulance. If I had booked them on a different plane they wouldn't have been on the one that crashed. If I had called them and delayed their departure ten minutes they wouldn't have been in that car wreck" and so on. If this type of guilt is not resolved it will activate the stress circuits, increase inflammation, and accelerate aging. But inappropriate guilt cannot be resolved by repentance and restoration because there is nothing to repent of or restore. Inappropriate guilt is resolved only by the application of the truth: "I wish I could have prevented their death, but there was nothing I could have done. Their death is not my fault." This type of guilt is often built on the hidden lie discussed above—believing one is responsible for how things turn out.

Another subtle form of the distortion that we are responsible for how things turn out, which causes false guilt, is the lie that we are responsible for how others feel, react, or think, that we are responsible for someone else's happiness—if they are not happy it is our fault. This is false. As stated above, we are responsible for making the healthiest choices in governance of self, not for how another person feels about those choices. A husband can buy his wife roses because he loves her, but he cannot cause her to enjoy the flowers and feel valued. If she is insecure she might instead feel doubt, and worry, "Why did he do this? Has he cheated on me and is he trying to offset his guilt with gifts?"

If you are experiencing guilt and would like to resolve it, then take the following three steps:

1. Ask yourself, Did I actually do something wrong?
2. If the answer is yes, then examine the wrong choice, repent, learn from the experience, forgive yourself, make a decision to act differently in the future, and if possible restore what was damaged or taken.
3. If the answer is no, then identify the lie, replace it with the truth, and set others free to think or feel as they choose.

Ongoing Relationship Conflict

Healthy relationships promote better health and longevity, but ongoing relationship conflicts undermine health and shorten life span.

As described in chapter 3, early childhood experiences impact brain development. When those early childhood experiences are traumatic, the brain's stress circuitry (amygdala) up-regulates and the braking mechanisms to calm the amygdala are impaired. Multiple studies have documented that healthy parent-child relationships reduce the risk of mental and physical illness and promote longer life. Children reared in homes with family conflict experience higher mental stress with higher rates of mental illness, obesity, diabetes, and inflammatory problems and die at a younger age than children raised in homes in which there is low conflict.[4]

Another recent study of nearly ten thousand men and women ages thirty-six to fifty-two examined how frequently they had conflict with their partners, children, friends, or neighbors and whether they worried about demands from their family. Eleven years later, 4 percent of the women and 6 percent of the men had died. Almost half the deaths were from cancer, the rest from heart disease, accidents, suicide, and liver disease from alcohol use. Those who had family conflict had 3 times higher risk of dying than those with low family conflict, and those who worried had 1.5 times higher risk of dying.[5]

The reason for this seems to be related to thought processes impacting the stress circuitry and either activating or calming it, with a subsequent effect on the immune response of either increasing or decreasing inflammation. This happens through multiple epigenetic pathways. Thus, healthy relationships can turn on antiinflammatory genes and shut down inflammatory ones.

A small pilot study examined gene expression in the white blood cells of six lonely people compared to eight socially connected people and found 209 genes were expressed differently. The researchers discovered that in the lonely individuals, genes associated with inflammation were up-regulated and viral-fighting genes were down-regulated.[6] This means the lonely individuals were more prone to infections and oxidative stress, with accelerated aging. Their findings were replicated in a larger study of ninety-three people.[7]

In a study published in *JAMA Psychiatry* in November 2016 researchers discovered an association between loneliness and the amount of amyloid (protein associated with increased risk for Alzheimer's dementia) deposited in the brain of cognitively normal older adults. After controlling for age, sex, genetic vulnerability to amyloid clearance (*ApoE4*), socioeconomic status, depression, anxiety, and social network, it was discovered that a higher amyloid concentration was significantly associated with greater loneliness. Those with high amyloid concentrations in their brain were found to be 7.5 times more likely to be in the lonely group.[8] This is likely due to the fact that loneliness increases the stress pathways, which increases inflammation and results in increased oxidative stress on the brain, contributing to more neuronal death and impaired repair mechanisms.

Healthy relationships require healthy people, so the first step to a healthy relationship is to do everything in your own power to be the healthiest person possible. Healthy people use their energies to benefit those with whom they relate, set healthy boundaries, speak honestly, allow others to wrestle with and overcome their life challenges and thus develop ever-increasing capacity and maturity, forgive those who do them wrong, and choose to extricate themselves from relationships that have proven to be toxic.

Finally, numerous scientific studies have documented the multiple health benefits from a spirituality that reduces fear and calms the stress circuitry. Documented benefits include reduced heart rate, blood pressure, and anxiety; improved depression; improved attention, concentration, and performance in school; as well as more rapid recovery from illness and less pain after surgery.[9]

The spiritual pursuits that consistently demonstrate health benefits are meditation with an emphasis on love, other-centeredness, compassion, and altruistic activities. Religious beliefs and practices that incite fear and anxiety are consistently demonstrated to be harmful.

The benefit of healthy spirituality occurs even when started later in life. Brain research by Dr. A. Newberg and colleagues at the University of Pennsylvania with individuals sixty-five years of age and older documented that those who meditated on a God of love for twelve minutes per day for just thirty days experienced growth in the love circuits of the brain (anterior cingulate cortex) as measured by MRI brain scans, lower heart rates and blood pressure (a measure of reduced stress), and 30 percent improvement in memory testing; meditating on angry- and wrathful-god concepts was not beneficial.[10] Managing one's stress in relationship to a loving higher power is healthy for the brain!

Integrating the loneliness research with that of meditation on a God of love, one could hypothesize that practicing altruistic love—helping others—would also be beneficial for health and perhaps slow the aging process. Amazingly, that is exactly what the research shows. Studies document that older adults who regularly volunteer in their communities (after accounting for variables such as education, baseline health, smoking, etc.) live longer; have less illness, disability, depression, and dementia; and stay out of nursing homes longer than those who did not volunteer.[11]

▪ LEARNING POINTS ▪

1. Unresolved mental stress activates inflammatory cascades, accelerating aging.
2. The big three mental stressors are chronic worry, unresolved guilt, and ongoing relationship conflict.
3. The worldview one holds impacts the ability to cope with an unknown future—belief in a punishing god undermines the ability to trust to a higher power what is out of one's own control.

▪ ACTION PLAN: THINGS TO DO ▪

1. Fulfill your own duties and responsibilities to the best of your ability.
2. Trust outcomes to your higher power (if you have difficulty with this, reevaluate your beliefs about your higher power and identify what undermines your ability to trust).
3. Forgive those who have wronged you and let go of bitterness and resentment.

4. Forgive yourself if necessary.

5. Resolve any unremitting guilt.

6. Evaluate the burdens you are carrying and determine which are your responsibilities and which are not; focus on the decisions that are yours to make in governance of yourself, surrender outcomes to your higher power, and leave others free to react as they choose.

7. Make the distinction between making mistakes and choosing evil, and give yourself permission to make mistakes and then learn from them.

8. Evaluate your relationships and make healthy relationship choices, which may include ending dysfunctional relationships.

13

Love and Death

Resolving One's Mortality

Because I could not stop for death—
He kindly stopped for me.

Emily Dickinson (1830-86)

The pain in her chest was crushing; sweat poured off her as she gasped for each breath. Her hands shook, waves of nausea rolled over her, and she was light-headed. She knew she was going to die. She was terrified, and she was in my office. The panic attacks had begun two months earlier—the day her father died in a car accident—and they had gotten worse with each passing day. She was consumed with fear—fear of death. She was a Christian and attended church each week, yet she was still afraid. And she is not alone; many of my patients, from all backgrounds, present to my office afraid of dying—worried, anxious, and insecure—desperate for some answer to bring them peace.

In his book *Existential Psychotherapy*, renowned professor of psychiatry Irvin Yalom writes:

"Don't scratch where it doesn't itch," the great Adolph Meyer counseled a generation of student psychiatrists. Is that adage not an excellent argument against investigating patients' attitudes toward death? Do not patients have quite enough fear and quite enough dread without the therapist reminding them of the grimmest of life's horrors? Why focus on bitter and immutable reality? If the goal of therapy is to instill hope, why invoke hope-defeating death?[1]

Yet how can we have a book on aging without considering the reality of our own mortality and the end of life as we know it? Yalom goes on to describe that the fear of death is universal, something with which all humans, from all backgrounds, struggle—a fundamental human reality: "The terror of death is ubiquitous and of such magnitude that a considerable portion of one's life energy is consumed in the denial of death."[2] And as we have discussed in previous chapters, unresolved fear from any cause increases activation of our stress circuitry with subsequent inflammatory cascades and accelerated aging. Further, if the fear of dying is significantly distressing it could lead to unhealthy coping, such as using alcohol or drugs, which would only accelerate decline. Therefore, for the healthiest aging we need to address the universal fear of dying.

Yalom is not the first to realize this universal fear of death. Almost two thousand years ago the writer of Hebrews wrote that one of the primary purposes of Christ's mission to earth was to "free those who all their lives were held in slavery by their fear of death" (Heb. 2:15). Christianity is not the only religion in which addressing concerns about death is integral. The ancient Egyptians were perhaps extreme in their concerns with death and the afterlife. They not only had an entire holy book focused on the mysteries of death but also spent vast fortunes in this life building incredible burial vaults (pyramids) and setting aside riches for the afterlife.

Nearly 30 percent of the world's population adheres to a religion that was founded because of one person's fear of death and his attempt to resolve that fear. Gautama Buddha lived between 563 and 483 BCE in the foothills of the southern Himalaya Mountains. As a young man, he left the confines of his luxurious apartments and encountered for the first time in his life a decrepit old man, a severely ill man, and a corpse being carried to the funeral pyre by mourners. Buddha realized that he was mortal, experienced fear of dying, and began a search to resolve his fear, which resulted in Eastern meditation practices and the development of Eastern philosophical explanations about life and death. These practices have continued and been developed and expanded by adherents over the millennia since Buddha died.

Most cultures of the world have faced the question of death and brought forth various beliefs to overcome and mitigate fears about it. Eastern religions address the fear of death through the recycling of life energy in a series of new lives (reincarnation), but most world religions have some form of heaven and hell. The Norse people believed that at death a person went to be with the various gods. If one died in battle one went to be with Odin, if drowned in the sea one went to be with the sea god, and so on.[3]

Zoroastrianism, an ancient religion from the Middle East, believes that at death each person must cross the Bridge of Judgment and is met by either a beautiful, sweet-smelling maiden or an ugly, foul-smelling old woman. If met by the young maiden one is taken to paradise; if met by the old woman one is taken to hell.[4]

Hinduism also believes in an afterlife, in the rebirth of souls into various planes of existence.[5] And within Islam the belief in both heaven and hell is accepted across all sects. The Koran has many texts that refer to the rewards in heaven for the faithful.[6]

Within Judaism there has been a historic divide, which became a point of great dissension during the time of Jesus Christ and in the first century following his crucifixion. The Pharisee sect (of which the apostle Paul was a member) believed in the resurrection of the dead, but the Sadducee sect did not. (Some remember the difference between the Pharisees and Sadducees on this issue by this mental witticism: the Sadducees did not believe in a resurrection so they were *sad—you—see*.) This divide in Judaism became a point on which the Sadducees famously sought to expose Jesus as ignorant and foolish. We have the encounter recorded in the book of Matthew:

> Later that day, the lawyers and theology professors from the school of the Sadducees—those who teach that there is no resurrection—came to question Jesus. They asked: "Wise Teacher, Moses instructed us that if a man dies without having children, then his brother is to marry the widow and have children for him. Well, we recently had a situation involving seven brothers: The oldest married and died without having children, so his brother married the widow. But he also died without having children, as did the third brother who married her, and the rest of them—right down to the seventh. Eventually, the woman herself died. Can you tell us, when the dead awaken to live again, whose wife will she be since she was married to all seven?"
>
> Jesus answered without hesitation, "Your entire question is flawed, because you understand neither what Scripture teaches nor God's power and methods. When those who sleep in the grave arise to life, it will be into God's heavenly kingdom, and they will be like the angels in heaven who neither marry nor are given in marriage. Regarding your speculation about the resurrection, you would have better conclusions if you remembered what God has said to you. God says: "I am"—not "I was"—"the God of Abraham, the God of Isaac, and the God of Jacob." He is not the God of the dead—those who no longer exist—but the God of the living. (Matt. 22:23–32)[7]

Since recorded history, humankind has faced death, and every culture of the world has developed beliefs about what happens after death. In fact, the victory over death is perhaps one of the most crucial theological beliefs within Christianity. The apostle Paul makes this point central:

> If there is no resurrection of the dead, then not even Christ has been raised. And if Christ has not been raised, our preaching is useless and so is your faith. More than that, we are then found to

be false witnesses about God, for we have testified about God that he raised Christ from the dead. But he did not raise him if in fact the dead are not raised. For if the dead are not raised, then Christ has not been raised either. And if Christ has not been raised, your faith is futile. (1 Cor. 15:13–17)

I think Paul was right about the futility of life here on earth if there is nothing beyond this current existence. For the Sadducees and the modern humanist who believe there is only this life and nothing beyond, there is little hope to offer when dealing with death and the loss of loved ones. But with so many divergent teachings about death and the afterlife, including the belief in no afterlife, things can be confusing. Does any evidence exist to support a belief in an afterlife? And is there any rational reason to believe that one view on what happens at death is any more reliable than any other view? Amazingly, our modern information science and our understanding of the difference between matter, energy, and information—material, power, and data—make one view much more likely than all the others.

According to the Bible human beings are tripartite: "Now may the God of peace himself make you completely holy and may your *spirit* and *soul* and *body* be kept entirely blameless at the coming of our Lord Jesus Christ" (1 Thess. 5:23 NET, emphasis added). Interestingly, computers are also tripartite and can serve as a very poignant object lesson. In order to have an operational computer, one needs hardware, software, and an energy source. Having only two of the three results in a computer that will not operate. All three are required for actual functioning.

Living (operational) human beings are composed of three parts—body, soul, and spirit—and all three components are needed for an *operational* or functional human being. The reason many people misunderstand this is because some biblical words have taken on magical or mystical meaning—for example, soul and spirit. Let's reexamine the New Testament Greek origins of these words and see if our understanding improves.

The Greek word for body is σῶμα, *soma*, from which the word *somatic* is derived. People who have mental stress that manifests in their bodies, such as stress ulcers, are said to have psychosomatic illness. *Soma* is our body, including our brain, and is analogous to a computer's hardware—the physical machine.

The Greek word for soul is ψυχή, *psuche*, from which we get *psyche* as in psychiatry and psychology. The Greek word means our unique individuality, personhood, and identity and is analogous to a computer's software.

And the Greek word for spirit is πνεῦμα, *pneuma*, from which we get *pneumonia* or *pneumatic* and which means wind, air, or breath—as in the breath of life. This is our energy source, the life energy originating from God.

To be operational a computer must have all three components— hardware, software, and an energy source. Likewise, to be *operational* a human being must have all three components—body (hardware), soul (software), and spirit (life energy).

When a computer runs out of power, into what state does it go? It "sleeps." Amazingly, this is the exact language the Bible uses for human beings who run out of power: they "sleep" (Pss. 7:5; 13:3; Matt. 9:24; John 11:12–13; 1 Thess. 4:13). And when our computer is "asleep" it is not dead; likewise, persons who enter this state that the Bible calls sleep are not dead. This is how Jesus could say that those who believe in him will never die—they may sleep, but they won't die (John 11:26).

What if someone were to take your computer and smash it into pieces and melt those pieces in a fire. You could at that point say they have "killed" or destroyed your machine. But what if your computer was backed up on the cloud? If that were the case, you could obtain a new piece of hardware and download the software from the cloud. What have you just done? You have resurrected your computer!

Jesus said, "Do not be afraid of those who kill the body [*soma*/ hardware] but cannot kill the soul [psyche/software]" (Matt. 10:28). Jesus is saying exactly what you would say to a friend whose computer is in the hands of an enemy threatening to destroy it but who knows a complete and perfect backup of their data is secure on the cloud. You would say, "Don't worry about those who can destroy the hardware but cannot destroy the software." Why? Because you can get new hardware (a hardware upgrade even) and download your software onto it; in the end, with the hardware upgrade, you will be in a better position.

This is what the Bible teaches: at the second coming of Christ the mortal puts on immortality and corruption puts on incorruption—we get hardware upgrades at the second coming (1 Cor. 15:42)! And our unique individualities, personhoods, and identities—our souls—are downloaded from God's heavenly servers (the Lamb's Book of Life) into our new bodies (hardware), and we become operational again!

Notice Paul's description and how he puts it all together:

> Brothers and sisters, we do not want you to be uninformed about those who *sleep* in death, so that you do not grieve like the rest of mankind, who have no hope. For we believe that Jesus died and rose again, and so we believe that *God will bring with Jesus those who have fallen asleep in him*. . . . For the Lord himself will come down from heaven, with a loud command, with the voice of the archangel and with the trumpet call of God, and *the dead in Christ will rise first*. After that, we who are still alive and are left will be caught up together with them in the clouds to meet the Lord in the air. And so we will be with the Lord forever. (1 Thess. 4:13–14, 16–17, emphasis added)

This is an incredible passage; here we have the dead in Christ coming down from heaven and at the same time coming up out of the graves. How is this possible? Because we are tripartite, at death the hardware/body (*soma*) returns to dust (Gen. 3:19; Job 34:15; Pss. 90:3; 104:29; Eccles. 3:20), the energy (spirit) returns to God (Eccles. 12:7), and the software/individuality (soul) is secure with Christ in heaven, safely stored on the heavenly servers—the

Lamb's Book of Life—awaiting the day our software (souls) gets downloaded into perfect hardware (bodies) and God breathes in the breath of life and the dead live again!

This is how Jesus could say, "I am the resurrection and the life. The one who believes in me will live, even though they die; and whoever lives by believing in me will never die" (John 11:25–26). Jesus had to speak a language they could understand. He had just told his disciples that Lazarus was asleep, but because they didn't understand he told them Lazarus was dead. Then Jesus says though a person dies they will never die. This could sound like a contradiction, unless one understands there are two deaths—one that we humans call death but God calls sleep and the other that God calls death and is the cessation of one's existence. Thus, Jesus is saying those who die (sleep) but trust in him will never die (cease to exist).

This is a great distinction between what Jesus taught and what Buddha taught. Jesus saw life energy (spirit/*pneuma*) and individuality (soul/*psyche*/software) as different. While energy cannot be created or destroyed but only transferred (in harmony with the first law of thermodynamics), information/data can be created and destroyed. Eastern religions merge life energy and individuality into one and teach that when life energy continues on in various forms so does the individuality that was using that energy. This teaching, however, is not consistent with either physics or information science. Incredibly, what the Bible writers describe is in complete harmony with modern science!

The entire emphasis of the Bible is that we are to receive new software here and now—we don't get new hardware until the second coming! The metaphors used in Scripture all teach this:

- Being reborn—not a new body or life energy but new motives, desires, priorities; new software, new *psyches*
- New heart—not a new body or life energy but new love, values; new way of viewing the world through the lens of love

- Circumcision of the heart—not a new body or life energy but new attachments, new affections, new heart bonds
- Eating the flesh and drinking the blood of Christ—not a new body or life energy but internalizing the word/truth from God and partaking of the perfect life of Jesus, thus experiencing a new operating system in harmony with Jesus
- Partaking of the divine nature—not a new body or life energy but the infusion via the Holy Spirit of Christ's perfect character of love, replacing our character of me-first, survival-of-the-fittest
- Having the law written on the heart and mind—not a new body or life energy but having God's methods, motives, ways of love, truth, and freedom replace the ways of fear, selfishness, and deceit in our operating systems

Christianity teaches that those who trust Jesus also open their hearts, and the Spirit comes in and transforms their souls/*psyche* (software), instilling new desires, motives, and methods of love while cutting out the ways of fear, selfishness, and evil. But all this happens in a defective and fallen body, which is slowly aging and decaying and will eventually wear out. When our bodies fail, the power runs down and they "fall asleep." But those who have trusted Jesus have their souls (individualities), which have been renewed to be like Jesus in character, safely secured with Christ in heaven, awaiting download into new bodies at the second coming!

We don't have to live in fear of death because our souls, our individualities, our software cannot be destroyed by any evil power on earth. Our souls—individual characters—can only be corrupted by us: by willfully participating in evil, by rejecting truth, by rejecting love, by choosing selfishness. But for those who choose Christ, who surrender self in trust to him, nothing can touch their software—their souls; their hearts are reshaped to be like God and are secure with him in heaven!

Unfortunately, for the good-hearted scientist who has rejected the dictator view of God and chosen to believe in a universe in which there is no afterlife, there is no protection from the fear of dying. Such people often try to offset their fear of no longer existing by having children (continuing to exist in their offspring), creating art or books that will continue to exist after they are gone, or leaving legacies (endowments, having buildings named after them, etc.). But all such attempts ultimately fail to bring genuine peace.

I would like to offer the open-minded scientist an alternative view—the belief in an intelligence who is perfectly kind, benevolent, and merciful and who constructed the very laws on which all the universe operates. Such a being desires thinking, inquiry, and forming of beliefs based on evidence, and for all who trust him he will secure their individuality for download into perfected hardware for eternity.

For the scientist who struggles with the language of the Bible, one could easily reword Genesis 1:1 from "In the beginning God created the heavens and the earth" to "Earth began when an extraterrestrial Intelligence came and terraformed it, establishing a viable atmosphere and a stable planet." Belief in a supreme intelligence who is love, who seeks to heal and restore, and whose laws are design parameters on which life is built allows for the integration of science and Scripture and provides a platform for refining our beliefs to conform ever more closely to how reality works. It also provides hope in a life to come that frees us from our fear of death. Such a belief reduces the firing of fear circuits and decreases inflammatory cascades, resulting in a healthier life here and now and a reduced risk of disability and dementia as we age. I invite you to consider this evidence for yourself.

▪ LEARNING POINTS ▪

1. Fear of death is a universal human concern with which all thinking people at some point grapple.

2. Materialism and theories promoting a godless universe offer nothing to address this concern and reduce anxiety.

3. Religions throughout history have taught a wide range of beliefs about death and what happens after death. Many of these beliefs are more fear inducing and less reasonable than the theory of a godless universe and have driven many people to reject the belief in a higher power.

4. Of the many religious views on death, the Christian view, with its teachings of a tripartite humanity (body/hardware, soul/software, spirit/energy), fits exactly the evidence of modern computer science.

5. A belief in a benevolent Creator, who constructed reality and who preserves human individuality (soul/software) on heavenly servers for future download into upgraded hardware (new bodies), is a reasonable hope consistent with a harmonized understanding of both the Bible and science.

▪ ACTION PLAN: THINGS TO DO ▪

1. Take a moment and answer the following questions:

   a. What do you believe will happen to you when you die?

   b. On what evidence do you base your answer?

   c. Does your answer bring peace or incite fear?

2. Formulate a belief system that is evidence-based and reduces anxiety and fear.

3. Choose to engage in activities that are altruistic, compassionate, and helpful to others.

4. In good conscience, refuse to engage in activities you know are harmful or that you would be ashamed of should they become public.

PART 4

PATHOLOGICAL AGING

14

Pathological Aging

Alzheimer's Disease (AD)

When people say, "You have Alzheimer's," you
have no idea what Alzheimer's is. You know it's
not good. You know there's no light at the end
of the tunnel. That's the only way you can go.
But you really don't know anything about it.
And you don't know what to expect.

Nancy Reagan, speaking to Mike Wallace
on *60 Minutes*, September 24, 2002

Dementia is not normal. Normal aging does not result in
dementia. Dementia is a pathological state—an abnormal
situation—a disease state that may, with healthy choices,
be avoided.

Dementia is the term for any condition that damages brain tissue
in such a way that there is permanent loss of memory along with
at least one other cognitive ability, such as the ability to problem

solve, organize, and plan; use language normally; identify common objects; or do simple motor tasks like buttoning a shirt or tying a shoe.

Dementia can be caused by head trauma (recently documented in football players but also boxers and individuals with any severe head injury), multiple strokes, infections (HIV, mad cow disease), or chronic metabolic problems that slowly destroy brain tissue (Alzheimer's disease). The term *Alzheimer's disease* refers to the neurodegenerative changes that occur in the brain. The term *Alzheimer's dementia* refers to the constellation of symptoms (memory loss and cognitive impairment) that are caused by the disease (damage to the brain). Thus, dementia can have many causes, the most common of which is Alzheimer's disease. But how common is dementia and what contributes to it?

Prevalence refers to the proportion of people in a society who have a condition at any given point in time. In most regions of the world 5–7 percent of those over sixty years of age have some form of dementia, with higher rates in Latin America (8.5 percent) and lower rates in sub-Saharan Africa (2–4 percent). In 2010 approximately 35.6 million people worldwide had some form of dementia, and numbers are projected to double every twenty years through 2050 (65.7 million in 2030, 115.4 million in 2050).[1]

In 2014 in the United States, it was estimated that 5.2 million people had Alzheimer's disease (AD), 5 million of them over the age of sixty-five and 200,000 under the age of sixty-five. One in nine persons over the age of sixty-five (11 percent) have AD, and almost one in three (32 percent) of those over eighty-five years of age have it. The vast majority of people with AD are over the age of seventy-five (82 percent). In America in individuals over the age of eighty-five, Hispanics have the highest rates of AD (62.9 percent), followed by African Americans (58.8 percent), and then whites (30.2 percent). Almost two-thirds of people with AD are women (3.2 million women, 1.8 million men). Of those seventy-one years old and older, 16 percent of women and 11 percent of men have AD.[2] One of the primary reasons for this gender difference is that women live longer than men, and as we have seen throughout this book, the longer a person lives the greater their risk for AD. But I want to emphasize again that living a long life does not mean one will get AD; it all depends on many modifiable factors in a person's life. One of the main goals of this book is to identify those factors so that people can make changes in their lifestyle that will not only increase length of life but also simultaneously reduce their risk of developing dementia.

What Is Alzheimer's Disease?

Alzheimer's disease was first described in 1907 by Alois Alzheimer, who identified the syndrome of memory and cognitive problems in a fifty-one-year-old woman whose autopsy revealed, under microscopic examination, lesions in the brain called *neurofibrillary tangles* and *senile plaques*. Neurofibrillary tangles are clumps of a specific protein called *tau* that has had excessive amounts of phosphate attached to it. The binding of phosphate to tau proteins impairs them from being able to do their normal job. Thus, they congregate together in these tangled masses observable in a biopsy.

Senile plaques are accumulations of a different protein, *beta*-amyloid (*b*-amyloid), which is thought to be a hallmark feature of and potential contributing factor in AD. As we will describe shortly, the buildup of tau and *b*-amyloid occurs when neurons die, thus neurofibrillary tangles and senile plaques are seen only in brains that have lost neurons. By the time a person has symptoms of AD their brain has already lost billions of neurons.

When the brain is operating normally it is in a state of flux with the production of new neurons, the elimination of unneeded neurons, and the constant branching and pruning of its axons and dendrites (the communication fibers that link neurons with other neurons and form vast networks for information processing).

This means that the brain has designed methods to eliminate and remove unneeded neurons in a controlled and nontoxic manner. This would be similar to how a demolition company collapses a building in a way to avoid damage to nearby structures. But in the aftermath of the collapse there is a lot of waste material left behind that needs to be cleaned up and removed.

When a neuron dies the various proteins, fats, and chemicals left behind need to be cleaned up. The brain has "crews" to do this. The immune system plays a role with some of the materials being "digested" by phagocytes. Other materials left behind such as copper, zinc, and iron can be very oxidizing and create reactive oxygen molecules that are damaging to the brain. The brain has a special protein designed to bind these trace chemicals and remove them. B-amyloid is the protein that binds these chemicals and then, normally, is quickly removed from the brain through the glymphatic system.[3]

Not only is b-amyloid involved in binding and removing trace chemicals, but it also, in very small amounts, could be necessary as a signaling molecule to trigger new neuronal growth.[4] However, if there is too much b-amyloid it can become toxic and contribute to the formation of destructive oxidizing molecules. Three events are required in order for b-amyloid to turn toxic. First, it must experience a structural change in which it folds back on itself and forms insoluble fibrils in a process called *fibrillation*. B-amyloid is normally a soluble protein, and as long as it remains in a soluble form the brain can excrete it and prevent a buildup. However, if b-amyloid misfolds into what are called *cross-sheets*, it then becomes insoluble and builds up in the brain, forming amyloid deposits.[5] The second event needed to turn b-amyloid toxic is the binding with copper or iron when cells die. And third is the presence of the amino acid methionine.[6] In fact, studies have shown that when b-amyloid increases in the brain without the presence of methionine there is a corresponding reduction in oxidizing molecules, which indicates that b-amyloid may be a compensatory mechanism working to reduce oxidizing molecules in the brain.[7] But when methionine binds to it, the clumps of *b*-amyloid begin generating oxidizing molecules that damage surrounding neurons. This would be analogous to sawdust used in a garage to absorb spilled gasoline. By absorbing the gasoline the sawdust reduces the ability of the gas to corrode other materials in the garage, and the two by themselves reduce damage in the garage. But if a third element is added, a spark, then combustion (which is rapid oxidation) occurs, causing increased damage to the materials in the garage.

So what is happening in the brain that contributes to Alzheimer's disease, and what can we do to reduce the risk or perhaps even prevent it?

There are two types of AD: early onset (before sixty-five, but more often before sixty) and late onset (sixty-five and older). Early-onset AD is genetically linked and known as Early-Onset Familial Alzheimer's Disease (EOFAD). Three genes have thus far been identified in EOFAD: *amyloid precursor protein* (*APP* on chromosome 21), *presenilin-1* (*PS1* on chromosome 14), and *presenilin-2* (*PS2* on chromosome 1). Mutations in any of these genes can cause EOFAD. *APP* mutations are associated with approximately 10–15 percent of EOFAD and *PS1* mutations are linked to 30–70 percent of EOFAD cases. *PS2* mutations are rare and contribute to fewer than 5 percent of early-onset AD.[8] Because EOFAD accounts for fewer than 5 percent of all cases of AD[9] and the primary risk factor is inherited, we will not explore this subtype further in this book.

Late-onset AD, which accounts for 95 percent of all AD, is associated with another gene, *ApoE*, which codes for a protein that transports fatty vitamins and cholesterol into the brain cells. In the human population three different versions of the gene that codes for *ApoE* have been identified: *ApoE2, ApoE3, ApoE4*. We have two sets of chromosomes—one received from our mothers and the other from our fathers—so that each person has two copies of *ApoE*.[10]

Seven percent of the population has at least one copy of the *ApoE2* gene, which increases their risk of atherosclerosis. This is when fatty plaques infiltrate the artery walls and narrow the width of the vessel, thus impeding blood flow and increasing the risk of heart attacks and strokes. Seventy-nine percent of the population has two copies of *ApoE3*, which is the healthy version and confers no known disease risk. Fourteen percent of people have at least one copy of the *ApoE4* version, which has been implicated in the increased risk of AD.

Persons with two copies of *ApoE4* have ten to thirty times the risk of developing AD, and up to 65 percent of people with AD have at least one copy of this gene. But one-third of people with AD do not have a copy of this gene, which means that while the *ApoE4* gene may increase the risk of developing AD, it is neither necessary nor sufficient on its own to cause the disease. When I first learned this good news I was so excited and relieved because it means that even if someone has the "bad" genes (often evidenced by family members suffering with late-onset AD), they can make choices that will prevent them from developing AD! Having a parent with AD does *not* mean you are condemned to getting it! There are choices you can make that will protect your brain and prevent AD from developing.

A recent study out of Washington University found that people with the *ApoE4* gene were not demented and had less *b*-amyloid in their brains *if they had a history of exercise!*[11] In this study, just one modifiable factor—exercise—prevented AD from developing in those with the *ApoE4* gene. And there are other modifiable factors as well that reduce the risk of developing AD. Genetics accounts for only about one-third of the risk of developing AD. What is the key, then, to developing AD if it isn't simply genetics? Strong evidence points to inflammation (the increase in oxidative molecules, cytokines, chemokines, and immune cells described previously), which contributes to insulin resistance in the brain and causes a cascade of events, resulting in the death of brain cells and the development of AD. Exercise, along with most of the other modifiable factors, reduces inflammation and insulin resistance, thereby preventing the development of AD.

Insulin and the Brain

In the body, insulin regulates glucose use and directs the body to store energy, primarily in the form of fat. When insulin levels are high the body is sent the signal to make fat and not to break down and burn the fat already stored. Insulin used throughout the body is produced by small clusters of cells called *islet cells* located within the pancreas.

But the brain makes its own insulin, and in the brain insulin does far more than just control glucose use. Within the brain insulin also regulates the clearance of b-amyloid protein and tau phosphorylation (remember that both of these are hallmark features of AD), blood flow, inhibition of cell death (apoptosis), response to inflammation, removal of fats from the brain, the ability of new synapses to form, and memory formation, and it facilitates neurotransmitter receptor trafficking.[12] As you can see, anything that interferes with insulin function in the brain will have wide-ranging negative effects.

There are striking similarities between AD and diabetes mellitus type 2 (T2DM), which is the adult-onset type that results from insulin resistance, not a lack of insulin in the body. In both AD and T2DM there is insulin resistance, inflammation with increased oxidative stress, b-amyloid protein deposits (in the brain in AD and in the pancreas in T2DM), hyperphosphorylated tau protein, and cognitive decline.

Having T2DM increases the risk of AD by 60 percent, and having elevated blood sugar (105–120 mg/dL) not yet severe enough to be diagnosed with T2DM increases the risk of AD by 10–20 percent.[13] This is quite alarming as 50 percent of Americans between the ages of forty-five and sixty-four have peripheral insulin resistance with normal blood sugar levels, and 76 percent of people older than sixty-five have peripheral insulin resistance. This means that inflammation is increasing in their bodies, causing insulin receptors to be less responsive to insulin. The body responds by increasing insulin levels to try to compensate, thus for a while glucose levels are normal. Factors that contribute to insulin resistance are anything that increases inflammation but specifically a high-fructose diet, a high-fat diet, chronic inflammation, chronic stress, and a sedentary lifestyle.[14]

The Destructive Cascade

In order to formulate a possible mechanism of what is going wrong, we need to understand a little more about neurons and their internal structure. Neurons are brain cells that have thousands of connections to other brain cells and communicate with electrical and chemical signals. Extending from the cell bodies of neurons are projections called *axons* and *dendrites*. These projections would be analogous to telephone wires that send (axons) and receive (dendrites) signals. It is through these projections that the neurons communicate with each other. Inside the axons and dendrites are microtubules, made of proteins called *tubulin*, which give them structure and stability and act as highways transporting vital materials around the inside of the cells. The microtubules in axons, but not dendrites, are held together by tau proteins.[15]

Consider a scaffold and how at each junction in the scaffold are pins that hold the joints together. The scaffold would be analogous to the microtubules, and the pins would be analogous to the tau proteins that hold the microtubules together. What would happen if someone pulled out the pins in the scaffold? It would collapse, and this is what happens when tau proteins get phosphorylated. When phosphate groups attach to tau it can no longer do its job of holding the microtubules together, and therefore the microtubules in axons fall apart. When this happens the axon loses integrity, various ions flow into the cell, and the neuron dies.

Now let's put this together to identify a potential pathway contributing to AD that fits the evidence. Anything that contributes to increased inflammation such as unhealthy diet (chaps. 5 and 6), toxic substances (chap. 7), sedentary lifestyle (chap. 8), sleep disorders (chap. 9), failure to mentally unwind (chap. 10), and chronic mental distress and unhealthy belief systems (chaps. 11, 12, and 13) will cause an increase in the concentration of inflammatory molecules circulating throughout the body and, thus, within the brain. These inflammatory molecules will cause the following destructive cascade:

- The insulin subreceptor on neurons becomes less responsive to insulin.
- Because insulin response is impaired, *b*-amyloid protein is not being cleared from the brain.
- B-amyloid then phosphorylates tau proteins on the microtubules.[16]
- The tau proteins disconnect and the microtubules disintegrate.
- The collapse of the microtubules causes loss of integrity in the axon, influx of various ions, and neuronal death.
- When neurons die they leave behind trace amounts of various chemicals such as copper, iron, and zinc. These chemicals are oxidizing and if not removed can trigger various damaging reactions in the brain, so the brain sends *b*-amyloid to bind and remove them.[17] Also, in an effort to prevent further neuronal loss, the brain may marshal in additional small amounts of *b*-amyloid.
- However, the brain that develops AD is in a chronically inflamed condition, with insulin resistance, so the *b*-amyloid is not removed effectively and therefore builds up and causes

more phosphorylation of tau, and the cycle continues, destroying more neurons and eventually causing dementia.

Another potential pathway could look like this:

- Brain injury—trauma or hypoxia—with subsequent neuronal loss.
- Trace chemicals left behind.
- Brain increases *b*-amyloid to both scavenge trace chemicals and potentially contribute to neuronal health.
- B-amyloid clearance is impaired.
- B-amyloid causes phosphorylation of tau proteins in axons.[18]
- Tau proteins disconnect from microtubules, and the microtubules collapse.
- Axons lose integrity, ions flow in, and neurons die, leaving behind more trace chemicals, and the cycle repeats.

In addition to this cascade, if the *b*-amyloid that is building up in the brain is exposed to methionine, then those deposits also become oxidizing engines that damage neurons and contribute to further neuronal loss.

Recommendations to Prevent Dementia

The good news is that for the vast majority of people, this destructive cascade is preventable, even in those who have begun to show mild worsening in memory and cognition. When healthy lifestyle changes are implemented, progression to dementia is halted![19]

We can break down the specific actions that promote health, slow aging, reduce dementia risk, and keep the brain young to four major keys: physical exercise, mental stimulation, stress management, and nutrition and lifestyle.

Physical Exercise

Please review chapter 8 for the science behind the benefits of exercise. But as a quick summary, exercise reduces the risk of dementia and slows aging because it decreases oxidative stress throughout the body, triggers the production of multiple proteins that promote brain health and the production of new neurons, increases the release of brain-produced mood elevators, improves insulin sensitivity, and promotes weight loss. There are no negative health effects to regular, nonexcessive exercise.

Recommendations for optimal exercise include:

- Consult your physician before starting a new exercise regimen.
- Always start with low intensity and increase slowly to avoid injury.
- Engage in exercises that are mentally enjoyable, and avoid exercises you dislike.
- Engage in moderate aerobic exercise five days per week, thirty minutes per day (ten-minute bouts) or vigorous aerobic exercise three days per week, twenty minutes per day.
  - On a scale of 0 (sitting) to 10 (all out), moderate = 5, vigorous = 7–8
- Strength train at least two days per week.
  - Eight to ten different exercises; at least one set of ten to twelve reps each
- Flexibility train two days per week, ten minutes per day.[20]

Mental Stimulation

Regular physical exercise causes the muscles to produce powerful anti-inflammatory cytokines that reduce inflammation. Physical exercise increases blood vessel growth in the brain, which improves oxygenation. Additionally, regular physical exercise causes the brain to produce proteins that stimulate the brain to make new neurons and that increase the growth of neuron-to-neuron connections. Therefore, physical exercise makes new learning easier! And using your brain is critical to maintaining its health. As we exercise the brain, it produces additional factors that not only keep it healthy but also will even create new networks corresponding to new learning. So include regular, mentally stimulating activities such as puzzles, Bible study, learning a new language or a new sport, music or art lessons, or taking a college class. Combining physical and mental stimulation seems particularly helpful, such as learning to waltz or tango or play ping-pong or tennis. Remember, if you don't use it, you will lose it—so exercise both brain and body regularly!

Stress Management

Stress management does not mean avoiding anything that is stressful but developing strategies for resolving stress and maintaining an internal state of peace and wellness. Failure to manage stress results in increased activation of stress circuits and inflammatory cascades that accelerate aging and increase the risk of dementia. Specific actions for reducing pathological stress include the following.

Forgive others. Forgiving those who have done us wrong calms the stress circuits and reduces inflammatory cascades. Forgiveness means letting go of resentment, bitterness, and grudges; it does not mean extending trust. We wisely trust only those who are trustworthy. Bitterness, resentment, and holding grudges are toxic and activate the brain's stress pathways. Failure to resolve such feelings results in increased oxidative stress and damage to physical, mental, and relational health. Forgiving those who have offended us does not mean that what they did was okay but relieves us of carrying the toxic emotions of anger and resentment everywhere we go.[21]

Develop healthy relationships. Relationship conflict activates the brain's stress circuits, which turns on the immune system, causing increased levels of inflammatory factors. People with chronic relationship problems have higher rates of mental and physical health problems. Healthy relationships require healthy people, and healthy people are in governance of themselves. This means that the mature evaluate the evidence of the health of others and make decisions in governance of self regarding whom we spend time with, how much credence we give their attitudes and desires, and when to extricate ourselves from relationships that have proven to be toxic.

Be a giver. Multiple studies have demonstrated that persons who are involved in any form of regular volunteerism have better physical health and lower blood pressure, take fewer prescription medicines, maintain independence longer in life, and have lower rates of dementia. Loving other people is healthy for the brain.[22]

Minimize theatrical entertainment. The brain cannot tell the difference between a real threat and a perceived threat. If you watch stressful television programming it will activate the brain's stress pathways, increasing inflammation throughout the body. Brain research has demonstrated that theatrical entertainment (but not education programming) alters the brain structure, resulting in underdevelopment of the prefrontal cortex (where we plan, organize, self-restrain, attend, have good judgment) and overdevelopment of the limbic system (where we experience fear and irritability). This imbalance increases the risk for attention problems as well as anxiety and mood problems, which increase the risk of dementia.[23]

Build a relationship with the God of love. Individuals with a healthy spirituality, meditating on a God of love, have reduced anxiety and stress and overall a more meaningful and satisfied life. Research shows healthy spirituality reduces rates of suicide, increases life-satisfaction scores, and generally results in healthier relationships and lifestyle. Healthy spirituality has multiple benefits:

- More likely to forgive and less likely to hold a grudge, thus reducing inflammatory cascades
- Development of prefrontal cortex and calming of fear circuitry
- Engagement in more altruistic activities
- Trusting outcomes to higher power with less worry
- Healthier lifestyle with decreased toxic substances
- Healthier relationships with better conflict resolution

However, there are unhealthy forms of worship with god constructs that incite fear, promote hostility, and foment conflict. All such belief systems are associated with increased anxiety, dread, and worry; relationship conflict; and a general sense of life dissatisfaction, all of which increase inflammation and are unhealthy for the brain.

A University of Michigan study examined the difference in benevolent versus vengeful God constructs in Muslim refugees from Kosovo and Bosnia, 60 percent of whom had post-traumatic stress disorder. Of the refugees, 77 percent practiced "negative" forms of prayer such as praying their enemies "would pay for what they have done." In other words, 77 percent sought God to act in vengeance on their enemies. Researchers found that Muslims with positive prayers, prayers of forgiveness and seeking for peace and resolution of hostilities, had high levels of optimism, hope, and healthy adjustment. But those who had vengeance and anger-related prayers experienced reduced levels of optimism, hope, and healthy adjustment.[24]

Nutrition and Lifestyle

You have probably heard the old adage, You are what you eat. There is much truth in this saying. What we eat provides the nutrients and building blocks from which the tissues of our bodies are made. Diets high in sugar and saturated fats increase inflammation and oxidative stress, which accelerate the aging process and the decline in brain function. Conversely, diets high in fruits, nuts, grains, vegetables, cold-water fish, and olive oil provide antioxidants and other vital nutrients, which reduce inflammation and slow the aging process. In general, the more highly processed the food, the less healthy and more damaging to the body and brain. Multiple studies reveal that a Mediterranean diet not only reduces risk of developing AD but also, when combined with other lifestyle factors as described above, prevents decline in those already showing early memory and cognitive impairments and those with the *ApoE4* at-risk gene.[25]

The International Conference on Nutrition and the Brain symposium held in Washington, DC, July 19–20, 2013, developed specific nutritional guidelines to promote brain health and reduce dementia risk. The seven guidelines that emerged are as follows:

1. Minimize your intake of saturated fats and trans fats. Saturated fat is found primarily in dairy products and meats. Trans fats are found in many snack pastries and fried foods and are listed on labels as "partially hydrogenated oils."

2. Vegetables, legumes (beans, peas, and lentils), fruits, and whole grains should replace meats and dairy products as primary staples of the diet.

3. Vitamin E should come from foods, rather than supplements. Healthful food sources of vitamin E include seeds, nuts, green leafy vegetables, and whole grains. The recommended dietary allowance (RDA) for vitamin E is 15 mg per day.

4. A reliable source of vitamin B_{12}, such as fortified foods or a supplement providing at least the recommended daily allowance (2.4 µg per day for adults), should be part of your daily diet. Have your blood levels of vitamin B_{12} checked regularly as many factors, including age, may impair absorption.

5. If using multiple vitamins, choose those without iron and copper and consume iron supplements only when directed by your physician.

6. Although aluminum's role in Alzheimer's disease remains a matter of investigation, those who desire to minimize their exposure can avoid the use of cookware, antacids, baking powder, or other products that contain aluminum.

7. Include aerobic exercise in your routine, equivalent to forty minutes of brisk walking three times per week.[26]

▪ LEARNING POINTS ▪

1. Normal aging does not result in dementia—dementia is an abnormal disease state.

2. Dementia has many causes; Alzheimer's is the most common.

3. The *ApoE4* gene can increase risk but is not sufficient by itself to cause AD.

4. Inflammation with insulin resistance in the brain contributes to the destructive cascade causing AD.

5. Activities that increase inflammation and insulin resistance and promote the development of AD include a sedentary lifestyle, sugary and fatty foods, chronic mental stress, overwork, and sleep deprivation.

6. Activities that decrease inflammation and insulin resistance and prevent the development of AD include mental and physical exercise, an anti-inflammatory diet, rest and sleep, and stress management.

▪ ACTION PLAN: THINGS TO DO ▪

1. Talk with your doctor about developing a sustainable exercise routine that includes forty minutes of aerobic exercise five times per week.

2. Engage in lifelong learning, mental stimulation, and thought development.

3. Establish regular sleep routines.

4. Make dietary changes to increase fruits, nuts, vegetables, and omega-3 fatty acids while reducing inflammatory foods that contain a high-sugar content, saturated fats, and trans fats. Saturated fat is found primarily in dairy products and meats. Trans fats are found in many snack pastries and fried foods and are listed on labels as "partially hydrogenated oils."

5. Engage in volunteer activities in your community.

6. Forgive any wrongs and resolve bitterness and resentment.

7. Evaluate theatrical entertainment and reduce the amount of time spent watching highly stressful programs and watch more educational or mirthful programs.

8. Resolve relationship conflict—even if it means setting boundaries with people who refuse to engage in healthy ways.

15

Vitamins and Supplements That Prevent Dementia

> The doctor of the future will . . . interest his patients in the care of the human frame, in diet and in the cause and prevention of disease.
>
> Thomas Edison, "Edison Hails Era of Speed,"
> *The Fort Wayne Sentinel*, December 31, 1902

As we saw in chapters 5 and 6, nutrition plays a critical role in our physical health and can accelerate aging or slow it, depending on whether we eat inflammatory foods devoid of essential nutrients (fast foods, junk foods) or a well-balanced diet filled with anti-inflammatory nutrients. Because this is a proven fact, millions of people seek to improve their health by augmenting their diets with nutritional supplements, various herbs, oils, vitamins, and minerals. It is estimated that Americans spend between $14 billion and $20 billion annually on various nutritional supplements—the majority of which have no evidence of benefit and some of which are even harmful. In this chapter we will review the data on supplements with the best evidence for promoting brain health and reducing risk of dementia.

Omega-3 Fatty Acids

In chapter 6 we examined some evidence for omega-3 fatty acids, noting that there are three omega-3 forms: a short-chain form (alpha-linolenic acid [ALA]) found in plants such as flax and nuts and two long-chain forms (eicosapentaenoic acid [EPA] and docosahexaenoic acid [DHA]) found primarily in oily fish. It is the long-chain forms (EPA/DHA) that the brain utilizes.

DHA is essential for healthy brain development, and deficiencies increase the risk of developmental delays.[1] Studies have found that children with low levels of these essential fats perform worse in school and have more behavior problems as compared to children with normal amounts.[2] This is one reason most obstetricians now include omega-3 supplements with prenatal vitamins. Because these fatty acids are essential to brain development, the mother's body will give omega-3s to the developing fetus during pregnancy, thus reducing her stores of this essential fat. This reduction in omega-3 fatty acids is one factor that increases the risk of postpartum depression and another reason for prenatal supplementation.[3]

Once the brain is developed omega-3 fatty acids appear to play an ongoing role in reducing inflammation by scavenging oxidizing molecules and having an anti-amyloid effect on the brain. In one study it appears these benefits reduced the risk of developing AD.[4] Another study that evaluated individuals without the *ApoE4* gene found that those eating fish two to three times per week reduced their risk of AD by 50 percent over four years.[5] In another study, which followed almost nine hundred people over nine years, researchers found that those with the highest DHA levels had a 47 percent reduction in developing AD.[6]

Interestingly, it appears that eating fish and taking fish oil supplements do not result in the exact same benefits. A meta-analysis of various studies showed that omega-3 supplements improved cognition and processing speed for those with mild cognitive impairment (symptoms before dementia occurs) but did not benefit those already demented and didn't prevent the development of dementia.[7] However, the ingestion of fish once per week was positively associated with larger brain volume, particularly in memory centers of the brain. In a study of 260 people who ate broiled or baked fish at least once per week researchers found that their brains had more gray matter than those who did not consume fish, and this benefit was independent of omega-3 fatty acid levels in their bodies.[8] Battered and fried fish would not be expected to provide benefit, and are most likely harmful, due to the advanced glycation end-products and other oxidizing molecules.

The benefit of fish consumption was demonstrated in another very rigorous study published in the *Journal of the American Medical Association* in 2016. In this study the researchers did postmortem evaluations on participants in the Memory and Aging Project that followed individuals from 2004 to 2013. Of the 554 deceased participants, 286 brain autopsies were included in the study. The mean age at death for those in the study was 89.9 years. Seafood intake was measured by regular questionnaires during the years prior to death. Various dementia-related abnormalities were assessed, including those associated with AD, Lewy body dementia, large strokes, and small strokes. Tissue concentrations of mercury were also measured. After adjusting for age, gender, education, and total nutritional energy intake, those who ate one or more meals of fish per week had significantly less Alzheimer pathology in their brains. They had lower amounts of amyloid plaques and neurofibrillary tangles (conglomerations of tau proteins). And this benefit was specifically for those with the *ApoE4* gene. Those with the highest genetic risk of developing AD had less AD pathology in their brain if they ate fish one or more times per week! Interestingly, fish oil supplements showed no statistical benefit with any pathological marker. Those with high ALA (plant omega-3) intake had lower risk of having large strokes.

There was a positive correlation between the amount of fish consumed and the concentration of mercury in the body, which means the more fish consumed the higher the mercury in the body. However, the mercury levels were not associated with any brain pathology. In other words, while the mercury levels were higher in those consuming fish, the higher levels were not sufficient to negatively impact brain health.[9] This is good news for those who would like to consume fish but who are fearful to do so because of concerns about mercury.

Even though in the study above the higher mercury levels in those who consumed the most fish were not associated with brain pathology, many people have legitimate concerns about eating fish. For cultural or religious reasons some are vegetarians; others are concerned simply because mercury is a known toxin and there is no way to be certain any given piece of fish is not contaminated with high levels of mercury. Therefore, some choose vegetarian sources for omega-3 fatty acids. For those who prefer a vegetarian source of the long-chain (EPA/DHA) omega-3 fatty acids, there are marine algae sources. In fact, algae are the source from which the fish get their omega-3 fatty acids. The question that has not been studied is whether there is benefit from ingesting the omega-3s directly from the ocean plant sources (algae).[10] My own hypothesis is that if this is ever studied it will show benefit.

The evidence is clear, long-chain omega-3 fatty acids (EPA/DHA) have multiple health-promoting effects that reduce inflammation, protect the brain, and lower the risk of dementia. Some of the mechanisms by which the omega-3s provide these healthy benefits are by scavenging oxidizing molecules, improving neural membrane fluidity, and altering gene expression.[11] Omega-3 fatty acids lower the gene expression of multiple pro-inflammatory genes, significantly reducing inflammation in the body.[12] This may be one reason those with the *ApoE4* gene showed benefit from regular fish consumption.

Omega-3s are also blood thinners. So individuals on blood thinners should consult with their doctor before consuming large amounts of these oils.

Recommendations: Ensure long-chain omega-3 fatty acids (EPA/ DHA) are part of your diet. The strongest beneficial evidence is for regular fish consumption; however, for vegetarians I would recommend supplements from algae high in EPA/DHA.

Ginkgo Biloba

Ginkgo biloba (GB) is a popular supplement touted for its memory and cognitive benefits. It comes from the leaf of the Maidenhair tree and is marketed over the counter in various formulations. GB has three identified active compounds: ginkgolides, bilobalides, and flavonoids. Ginkgolides are believed to have anti-inflammatory effects and to help reduce blood clotting and improve blood flow. Bilobalides are thought to also reduce blood clotting, but in addition they reduce the activity of a neurotransmitter called *glutamate*. Glutamate is the brain's primary excitatory neurotransmitter. This means that glutamate is the most common agent in the brain to activate neurons and promote signaling. In proper amounts this is essential for thinking, learning, and memory. However, when glutamate levels are too high in the neural junctions (synapses) it creates noise that impairs clear signaling, thus reducing communication and impairing learning and memory. It would be similar to a radio station broadcasting on a specific frequency. When one station broadcasts, the signal is clear and communication is effective. But if multiple stations broadcast on the same frequency, there are too many signals coming in at once and communication is impaired.

As we discussed in chapter 14, the brain is capable of changing its structure based on use. It can grow new neurons and pathways and delete unused ones. This means that in a controlled fashion the brain has a mechanism to cause cell death. Glutamate is involved in this process. It triggers calcium channels to open and, by flooding the inside of the neurons with calcium, causes the cell to die. Thus, excessive glutamate not only impairs signaling and learning but also can cause neuronal death. One of the potential benefits of GB, therefore, is to reduce the activity of glutamate.

Finally, the flavonoids function as antioxidants, scavenging free radicals and thus reducing oxidative damage to the brain.[13]

Overall, most studies show that GB does provide memory and cognitive benefit in those who *already* have memory and cognitive disorders such as AD. There is little evidence that GB provides any improvements in memory and cognition in those who are cognitively unimpaired.[14]

Does GB have protective effects and reduce the risk of developing AD? The data is mixed. A study of three thousand people over seventy-five years of age failed to show any protective effects of GB in preventing dementia.[15] Another study evaluating the preventative effects of GB in people ages seventy-two to ninety-six with either normal cognition or mild cognitive problems over a six-year time period also found no reduction in risk of developing dementia from using GB.[16] In a large twenty-year study GB did show that it prevented dementia. However, the study was poorly documented with no GB dosage or duration of treatment recorded.[17]

It is difficult to compare findings from random-controlled trials and epidemiological studies (surveys of the population) because the epidemiological studies do not control for confounding variables. Overall, the evidence currently supports the use of GB for those who already have memory and cognitive impairments, but not for use as a preventative measure. Further, there appears to be no memory or cognitive benefit for individuals who are cognitively unimpaired. GB should be used with caution in those at risk for bleeding as it can act as a blood thinner, but studies have found it can be used safely alone or in patients on aspirin.[18]

Recommendations: Do not use ginkgo biloba as a preventative agent. It may be used if an individual is already experiencing memory and cognitive deficits; gauge continued use by response and any side effects.

Vitamin D

Over the last couple of decades research on the benefits of vitamin D has significantly increased, and the role of vitamin D in brain health has become clear. It appears vitamin D has a therapeutic window. This means that low levels of vitamin D contribute to a variety of health problems and early death,[19] but levels too high also contribute to health problems (such as bone fractures)[20] and early death.[21] Studies differ on what levels of vitamin D are optimal, but all agree that blood levels below 25 nmol/L (this is the concentration measured in the blood and how the lab will report it to your doctor) are unhealthy and confer greater risk of mental health problems and early death, and blood levels above 140 nmol/L are associated with early death. In addition to mortality risks, low vitamin D levels increase the risk of mental decline and dementia. In fact, those with vitamin D levels below 25 nmol/L had 2.22 times the risk of developing dementia as compared to those in the normal range.[22] A study of 1,927 older adults followed for 4.4 years found the highest risk for cognitive decline in individuals with vitamin D levels below 50 nmol/L and mild decline in those with levels between 50–75 nmol/L. This means that levels below 75 nmol/L are associated with increased risk of loss of cognitive abilities.[23] Therefore, according to these studies, an optimal level would be between 75–100 nmol/L.

The proposed mechanism by which vitamin D reduces the risk of dementia is by activating the macrophages, the trash cleaners of the body, to ingest and remove *b*-amyloid protein deposits from the brain.[24] If you remember from the chapter on pathological aging, *b*-amyloid is a protein that normally helps remove oxidizing trace chemicals such as copper and iron from the brain, but in AD it becomes fibrillated and builds up in the brain and can then begin damaging brain cells. Thus, clearing it from the brain has significant potential benefit.

Recommendations: Have your vitamin D level checked by your physician and take supplements as needed to achieve a level between 75–100 nmol/L.

Curcumin (Tumeric)

Curcumin is a yellow spice commonly used in Indian foods and has a long history of use in Eastern traditional medicine. It is known to have anti-inflammatory and antioxidant benefits, which is consistent with most edible plants that contain color. More recent lab studies noted that curcumin binds to amyloid protein and prevents its fibrillating,[25] which kept the amyloid in a soluble form and suggests it would reduce deposits in the brain. Animal studies confirmed that curcumin did reduce amyloid and tau deposits in the brain. In human studies on individuals already diagnosed with AD curcumin showed no benefit in memory or cognitive function.[26] This is likely due to the fact that by the time someone is diagnosed with AD the brain is already severely compromised with billions of cells lost. If curcumin has a benefit it would be in the preventative phases to help remove the buildup of amyloid from the brain and potentially reduce the cascade of events leading to accelerated neuronal death.

Evidence that curcumin might provide preventative benefits includes its known anti-inflammatory properties and its ability to help clear amyloid and tau proteins from the brain.[27] Additionally, it has been reported that people ages seventy to seventy-nine living in India have a 4.4–fold lower rate of AD than people living in America—suggestive, but not proof, that a diet rich in curcumin might confer benefit.[28] Lab studies have revealed that curcumin can bind copper and iron; if this occurs in the brain it would further reduce the oxidative damage from these trace chemicals.[29] Curcumin is a very powerful free-radical scavenger, which can reduce damage to the neuronal membranes.[30] And there are a host of other beneficial effects upon the brain that may reduce the risk of AD.[31] Very few outcome studies examining the clinical impact of curcumin on human populations have been done. One trial did show curcumin reduced both triglycerides and plasma b-amyloid levels.[32]

Curcumin has been shown to be well tolerated with little or no adverse effects. One problem with dietary curcumin is that very little is absorbed into the body; thus, taking supplements of curcumin would seem to provide little benefit. However, studies have documented that black pepper, which contains piperine, increases the absorption of curcumin by 2,000 percent.[33]

Recommendations: Use curcumin in a variety of dishes and be sure to add black pepper in all preparations.

Walnuts

Adults who eat walnuts regularly have significantly better cognitive ability than those who do not. In a cross-sectional study published in the *Journal of Nutrition, Health and Aging*, researchers examined the link between walnut consumption and cognitive abilities in areas such as memory, concentration, and processing speed. They examined two age groups, twenty-nine to fifty-nine and sixty and older. Researchers reported, "Significantly better outcomes were noted in all cognitive test scores among those with higher walnut consumption."[34]

This is certainly an interesting and encouraging finding, but why would researchers even think to look for a relationship between walnut consumption and cognitive performance? Because in 2004 other researchers discovered that walnut extract prevented b-amyloid from fibrillating—remember fibrillation is when this protein folds on itself, clumps together, and cannot be removed and therefore builds up in the brain. These clumps of *b*-amyloid, if bound with trace chemicals (iron and copper) in the presence of methionine, become little engines of destruction, contributing to increased oxidation and the phosphorylation of tau, which destabilizes microtubules and contributes to the death of neurons. So it would be beneficial to prevent the clumping of *b*-amyloid. But researchers found that the walnut extract did even more—it dissolved the amyloid clumps that had already formed! In other words, in this study the walnut extract not only prevented the clumps from forming but also defribillized the fibrils of amyloid already formed.[35] This research has led to the hypothesis that walnut consumption will decrease amyloid deposits in the brain and thereby reduce neuronal loss and provide cognitive benefit—something that seems to have been demonstrated to be true in the cross-sectional study cited above.

Recommendation: Eat a handful of raw walnuts daily.

Green Tea

Do you drink green tea? Perhaps you should consider it. Green tea is rich in antioxidants and flavonoids and studies demonstrate that those who drink it regularly have improved memory and cognition—even in those who have already demonstrated impairments.[36] One beneficial effect of green tea is that it reduces *b*-amyloid buildup in the brain.[37] Other research has demonstrated that higher green tea consumption results in decreased prevalence of cognitive problems in older adults.[38] What is interesting about green tea is that it appears to not only prevent cognitive and memory decline but also improve performance in those with no deficits.[39]

These various studies demonstrate that green tea appears to have several benefits: slowing decline, improving performance in those with deficits, and improving performance in those without deficits. This suggests that green tea may have multiple mechanisms of action that contribute to its benefits. And research has documented this to be true.

One action of green tea is its antioxidant action, reducing oxidative damage. Another is its ability to clear amyloid. Both of these actions would explain some of its ability to prevent cognitive decline and how it possibly could contribute to cognitive improvement in those already showing some deficits. But these actions don't explain why green tea enhances cognition in cognitively intact individuals. This led researchers to examine the effect of green tea on brain function, and they found very amazing results.

Functional brain-imaging studies reveal that the ingestion of green tea enhances neural activity and signaling in the part of the brain with which we reason, think, problem solve, and have working memory.[40] What is happening is that green tea appears to improve the communication pathways between the various brain regions, allowing the thinking circuits of the brain to have quicker and easier access to the various brain regions in which memories and experiences are stored.[41] All this research led brain scientists to examine whether green tea could actually cause neuronal connections to improve efficiency of signaling between frontal and other brain regions, allowing for better cognition and memory. And according to the researchers: "Our findings provide first evidence for the putative beneficial effect of green tea on cognitive functioning, in particular, on working memory processing at the neural system level by suggesting changes in short-term plasticity of parieto-frontal brain connections."[42]

Recommendation: Consume green tea on a regular basis.

Pomegranate Juice

Pomegranate juice contains higher concentrations of antioxidant polyphenols than most other juices. This led researchers to wonder if this juice may provide antioxidant protection to the brain and perhaps even prevent *b*-amyloid buildup in the brain. In order to investigate this hypothesis researchers used genetically modified mice. These mice were genetically engineered to have higher than normal amounts of *b*-amyloid deposits in their brains. The mice were randomized into two groups and both fed the same diet, except the experimental group received the human equivalent of eight ounces of pomegranate juice per day. Results showed that the mice who received the pomegranate juice not only learned faster and performed better on various tests but also had significantly less buildup of *b*-amyloid in the memory circuits of their brains.[43]

While this study was done on mice and has not been replicated in humans, it is consistent with epidemiological research in human populations done by researchers at Vanderbilt University. In a study examining the relationship between the consumption of fruit and vegetable juices and the development of AD, researchers found that those who consume three or more servings of juice per week were 76 percent less likely to develop AD as compared to those who ingested fewer than one serving per week. This protective benefit of drinking juice was even more pronounced in those who had the at-risk *ApoE4* gene. Researchers believed these benefits were due to the polyphenol content in the juices and not the vitamins, such as vitamins C and E, contained in the juices, as no benefit was demonstrated from supplements of vitamins alone.[44]

The Vanderbilt researchers' conclusion that the antioxidant benefit from the juices was due to polyphenols and not the vitamins was supported by later research that examined the antioxidant benefit of pomegranate juice versus apple juice in older adults. In this study twenty-six older adults were randomized into two groups and assigned to drink eight ounces of either apple juice (low antioxidant) or pomegranate juice (high antioxidant) for four weeks. The researchers measured blood antioxidant capacity and levels of antioxidant enzymes as well as levels of vitamins C and E and other molecules. Additionally, researchers examined DNA damage in white blood cells. Researchers found that the group drinking daily pomegranate juice demonstrated significantly improved antioxidant activity while those drinking apple juice did not. Plasma levels of vitamins C and E did not differ between the two groups, supporting the likelihood that the benefit from pomegranate juice was due to its high polyphenol levels.[45]

A more recent animal study examined the potential mechanism by which pomegranate juice may be neuroprotective. In this study researchers used mice genetically modified to deposit amyloid into their brains, which mirrors AD pathology. The mice were randomized into two groups with both having access to the same diet, but the experimental group had their water augmented with pomegranate juice. Both groups of mice were given standardized maze tests, which tested learning and memory. After three months of receiving pomegranate juice the experimental mice demonstrated significant improvements in navigating the maze as compared to their initial scores and their control-fed counterparts. Their brains had lower levels of inflammatory factors (tumor necrosis factor alpha [TNF]) and lower nuclear factor of activated T-cell (NFAT) transcriptional activity. This means their brains had fewer molecules that cause oxidative damage in the brain. Additionally, upon microscopic examination of the brains of the mice receiving pomegranate juice it was found that their brains had fewer clumps of white brain cells and b-amyloid. The researchers identified two polyphenol components of pomegranate juice, punicalagin and ellagic acid, that reduced the activity of NFAT and decreased the b-amyloid secretion of TNF. Researchers concluded: "These data indicate that dietary pomegranate produces brain anti-inflammatory effects that may attenuate AD progression."[46]

Recommendation: Drink one eight-ounce glass of 100 percent pomegranate juice per day.

Coffee

When I began this book I had certain biases—expectations that I assumed to be true due to my upbringing and previously held beliefs. I was raised not to drink coffee or other caffeinated drinks and taught that these drinks were unhealthy and should be avoided. Therefore, I was surprised to discover that caffeine functions much more like a medicine than the other substances discussed in this chapter, meaning that while it does have risks and side effects, it also has some significant benefits. We will discover that in certain individuals with known health problems caffeinated coffee intake can contribute to worsening health. In others, however, evidence demonstrates marked health advantages, including a significantly reduced risk of developing AD!

A large study published in the *New England Journal of Medicine*, which followed more than fifty thousand men and women for thirteen years, found that, after adjusting for other risk factors such as smoking, regular coffee consumption reduced all-cause mortality (risk of death). Specifically, those who regularly consumed coffee had reduced risk of dying from heart disease, respiratory disease, stroke, injuries and accidents, diabetes, and infections, but not cancer.[47] In a different study researchers reviewed articles published between 1990 and 2012 that examined coffee consumption and health impact and found that regular coffee consumption is also associated with reduced risks of a variety of diseases, including diabetes, liver disease, and Parkinson's disease.[48]

Some might wonder how a substance that can transiently increase blood pressure, as caffeine does, can reduce risk of death from cardiovascular disease (CVD) when high blood pressure is a known risk factor for CVD. The reason is likely because the increases in blood pressure from coffee are small and transient and therefore clinically insignificant, while at the same time coffee contains antioxidants that reduce low-density lipoprotein (LDL) cholesterol and prevent it from oxidizing and building up in arterial walls, as well as reducing other markers of inflammation.[49] In fact, in one ten-year study moderate coffee consumption (one to four cups per day) showed reduced heart disease risk during the entire study period;[50] other research revealed that coffee consumption reduces the risk of heart failure.[51]

The benefits of coffee consumption are not restricted to the heart. Stroke risk is also reduced by regular coffee consumption. A 2011 meta-analysis found that regular, moderate coffee consumption (one to six cups per day) reduced the risk of stroke by 17 percent.[52] And a study of Swedish women who were followed for ten years found that regular coffee consumption reduced strokes by 22 to 25 percent.[53]

Regular coffee consumption also appears to reduce the risks of type 2 diabetes (T2DM), obesity, high cholesterol, and high blood pressure—what are commonly called *metabolic syndrome*. Numerous studies have demonstrated that regular coffee consumption improves glucose metabolism and insulin secretion and reduces T2DM.[54] One reason for this may be coffee's effect on b-amyloid.

It is known that in T2DM, b-amyloid (the same protein that builds up in the brain in AD) is known to misfold (fibrillate) and build up in the cell clusters (islet cells) in the pancreas that secrete insulin. This buildup is believed to be one factor that impairs glucose metabolism and contributes to T2DM. Coffee extracts have three identified active components: caffeine, caffeic acid (CA), and cholorogenic acid (CGA). CA and CGA have an active metabolite (a new molecule that is produced when they are metabolized) called *dihydrocaffeic acid* (DHCA). All these components have been shown to inhibit the misfolding of amyloid and thereby reduce its toxic buildup in the pancreas. CA showed the greatest potency and caffeine the least potency in preventing amyloid misfolding.[55]

While the *New England Journal of Medicine* study mentioned above did not find reduced mortality from cancers associated with coffee consumption, other studies have found reduced risk of developing multiple cancers in moderate coffee drinkers. Studies reveal reduced cancer risk for endometrial cancer for those who drank four cups per day,[56] for prostate for those who drank six cups per day,[57] for head and neck (four cups per day),[58] for basal cell carcinoma (three cups per day),[59] and for estrogen receptor-negative breast cancer (five cups per day).[60] These benefits are thought to be at least partially due to the anti-inflammatory and antioxidant effects of coffee.[61]

As amazing as all these potential benefits of coffee are, the most important findings for this book are the effects upon the brain and the evidence that coffee not only enhances cognition and memory but also actually reduces the risk for AD. In a study published in the *Journal of Alzheimer's Disease* researchers found that those who consumed moderate daily coffee (three to five cups per day) at midlife decreased their risk of dementia by 65 percent later in life.[62] Additional research found that individuals who are already experiencing mild cognitive impairment but had high-plasma caffeine levels due to drinking three to five cups of coffee per day avoided progressing to dementia over the next two to four years.[63]

These benefits are likely due to the same anti-amyloid and anti-inflammatory benefits from coffee that provided benefit in reducing metabolic syndrome. In studies of mice genetically altered to mimic AD, the animals that received caffeine in their drinking water from young adulthood through older age showed protection from memory loss and had lower levels of *b*-amyloid in their brains than the mice without the caffeine. Not only that, but mice that were allowed to develop memory problems and amyloid deposits in their brains exhibited memory restoration and reduction of amyloid in their brains after one to two months of caffeine treatment. The researchers concluded the benefits were due to the caffeine itself, as animals that received caffeinated coffee demonstrated the benefit while the animals that received decaffeinated coffee did not. The benefits were achieved with the human equivalent of moderate coffee consumption (five cups per day).[64]

But it appears that it is not caffeine alone that provides the benefit. Other research suggests that the benefits to the brain result from a combination of the caffeine and other active compounds found in coffee. In this study of AD mice, researchers examined the effects of caffeinated versus noncaffeinated coffee on plasma cytokines (granulocyte-colony stimulating factor [GCSF], IL-10, IL-6), comparing the results to that of caffeine alone. In both the AD mice and the non-AD comparison mice researchers found treatment with caffeinated coffee greatly increased anti-inflammatory cytokines, whereas neither caffeine alone nor decaffeinated coffee demonstrated this positive effect. The increase in GCSF was thought to be particularly important because this compound among all those measured was most specifically associated with improved cognitive performance. The researchers concluded that "coffee may be the best source of caffeine to protect against AD because of a component in coffee that synergizes with caffeine to enhance plasma GCSF levels, resulting in multiple therapeutic actions against AD."[65]

The idea that coffee may be the best source of caffeine to provide neuroprotective benefits is supported by other research that examined various caffeinated drinks and their impact on mental health. The National Institutes of Health–AARP Diet and Health study, which was a prospective study of over five hundred thousand people ages fifty to seventy-one followed over ten years, found differences between soft drinks, fruit drinks, and coffee and the rates of depression. Those who drank soft drinks and fruit drinks had increased risk of developing depression, while those who drank coffee had slightly lower risk. Additionally, when they evaluated sweeteners they found that artificial sweeteners increased the risk of depression whereas sugar and honey did not. As little as one soft drink per day increased the risk for depression, regardless of whether the soft drink was caffeinated or decaffeinated. Decaffeinated teas were associated with slight increased risk of depression; however, caffeinated teas were not. Hot caffeinated tea had no relationship with depression and caffeinated iced tea had a weak decreased association with depression.[66]

This association with depression is an important finding because one of the primary factors contributing to depression is inflammation, which is the same underlying problem driving AD.[67] And research shows that a history of depression increases the risk for AD later in life.[68]

In addition, the neuroprotective benefits of coffee found to reduce risk of AD have also been associated with reducing the risk of Parkinson's disease (PD). But in the case of PD, researchers have identified specific gene variants in people who are at risk for PD that coffee specifically interacts with to reduce the risk of PD. A gene that regulates brain signaling that controls movement (*GRIN2A*) has been found to have more than one form in humans. Researchers found that heavy coffee drinkers with one gene variant had an 18 percent lower risk for PD compared to light coffee drinkers, whereas heavy coffee drinkers with another variant of the same gene had a 59 percent lower risk for PD compared to light coffee drinkers. The researchers emphasized that drinking coffee reduced risk of PD only in those with the specific gene variants.[69]

So what does all this mean? Caffeinated coffee appears to have an overall health-promoting benefit due to a combination of caffeine and antioxidant compounds working together. These benefits include reducing oxidizing chemicals and preventing amyloid from misfolding and building up in both the brain and pancreas, thereby reducing risk of T2DM, CVD, obesity, and AD. Other caffeinated beverages, with the exception of tea, most likely increase risk of health-related problems, while tea is either neutral or has a very slight positive effect. Natural sweeteners such as sugar and honey in beverages were not associated with increased mental health risks, whereas artificial sweeteners did increase risks for mental health problems.

There are several cautions when it comes to caffeine consumption that must be taken into consideration. Caffeine decreases seizure threshold, which means it increases the likelihood of having a seizure; for those with known seizure disorder, drinking beverages with caffeine may undermine seizure control.[70] In fact, caffeine is so good at increasing seizures that when doctors desire to lengthen seizures in patients receiving electroconvulsive therapy (ECT) for depression, they will give IV caffeine.[71] Individuals with seizure disorders should be very cautious about consuming beverages with caffeine.

Additionally, for some individuals caffeine can delay sleep onset and reduce total hours of sleep. There is wide variation to the sleep response of caffeine from person to person. Some individuals may have marked sleep impairment from mild to moderate caffeine consumption. If so, those individuals should limit caffeine because, as we discussed in chapter 9, sleep is a physical requirement to life and health, and chronic sleep disturbance increases risk of dementia.

Finally, caffeine is also a vasoconstrictor and has been demonstrated to reduce blood flow to the brain, the retinas, and throughout the body.[72] Therefore, health conditions with known circulatory compromise (CAD, macular degeneration, Raynaud's, etc.) may be worsened by caffeine use.

Recommendations: Drink one to six cups of caffeinated coffee per day (as long as sleep remains at 7–8 hours per night, no known circulatory or seizure risk factors exist, and no other intolerable side effects manifest). If desired, use sugar or honey to sweeten and avoid artificial sweeteners and all soft drinks. I personally use maple syrup as a coffee sweetener as recent research has documented that maple syrup not only has anti-inflammatory benefits but also reduces the aggregation of both *b*-amyloid and tau proteins.[73]

Vitamins E and C

Vitamin E supplementation as a medical strategy has had a rocky history. Early studies demonstrated vitamin E had antioxidant properties and could inhibit the oxidation of bad cholesterol and its buildup in arteries (atherosclerosis).[74] Some studies even showed that the higher the plasma vitamin E level, the lower the risk of dying of heart disease.[75] Other studies also noted an association with higher vitamin E and reduced cardiovascular disease risk.[76] Additionally, observational data also seemed to indicate that vitamin E supplementation reduced cancer risk.[77] Because of these observations, randomized clinical trials were undertaken to specifically examine and measure the effect of vitamin E supplementation. However, these various studies demonstrated no reduction in cardiovascular disease, cancer, or mortality from vitamin E supplementation.[78] Further, a meta-analysis of high-dose vitamin E supplementation found an increased risk of dying in those taking the supplemental vitamin E.[79] So what is going on with vitamin E?

Vitamin E occurs in nature in eight different forms divided into two classes, tocopherols and tocotrienols. When one ingests vitamin E from food one receives all eight forms. However, many over-the-counter vitamin E supplements have not provided the same natural balance. This difference may account for the variation in benefit noted in the various studies. For instance, in studies examining those with high vitamin E from dietary sources investigators found reduced risk of vascular disease and risk of death.[80] But in studies where supplements were used no health benefit was found.[81]

Animal studies support the benefit of *dietary* vitamin E on reducing the risk of AD. Vitamin E is a fatty vitamin, which means it will concentrate in the fatty tissues of the body. Within the brain this would be the lipid membranes of the neurons. Neuronal membrane health is critical to overall cellular health, as the membranes separate the internal machinery of the cells from outside forces. The membranes also act as gatekeepers regulating the flow of various molecules and compounds in and out of the cell and as filters keeping out potentially harmful substances. Vitamin E serves a critical role in this protective function. Vitamin E concentrating in the lipid membrane serves as a free-radical scavenger preventing these damaging molecules from entering the neurons and causing injury. Additionally, vitamin E in younger animals prevented the buildup of *b*-amyloid protein in the brain.[82] Two prospective studies in human populations have shown that dietary vitamin E lowers AD risk.[83] However, vitamin E *supplements* showed no benefit in reducing AD in human studies.[84]

Another factor in vitamin E's effectiveness may be the relationship between vitamins E and C. While E is fatty and concentrates in the lipid membrane, vitamin C is water-soluble and concentrates in fluid inside the cells. Vitamin C is a powerful antioxidant and plays a direct role in scavenging free radicals and reducing oxidative stress, and vitamin C has a number of other functions acting as a coenzyme in many critical pathways.[85] Additionally, vitamins E and C work together to protect the brain from oxidative damage. As free radicals try to enter the neuron, vitamin E in the lipid membrane works to scavenge and remove them; if free radicals make it past the lipid membrane, then vitamin C acts to inactivate it. But vitamin C also works to reactivate the antioxidant properties of vitamin E.[86] Studies demonstrate that vitamin C provides health benefits from both dietary and supplemental sources.

Recommendations: Get vitamin E from food sources, not supplements (recommended foods with the highest-to-lowest concentration of vitamin E include sunflower seeds, almonds, spinach, safflower oil, pumpkin, red pepper, asparagus, collard greens, and peanut butter).

Vitamin C from food or supplements should be 500–1,000 mg per day.

N-Acetyl Cysteine

N-acetyl cysteine (NAC) is an antioxidant that has been used to treat acetaminophen overdose for over thirty years. Recently, NAC has been shown to play a significant role in promoting and maintaining the brain's antioxidant defenses. One of the brain's primary antioxidant agents is glutathione, which directly and indirectly neutralizes both reactive oxygen and nitrogen molecules. In this role glutathione maintains the oxidative balance within cells and is highly concentrated in the white cells of the brain, which provide protection and support to the neurons. NAC is a direct precursor to glutathione and thus supplemental NAC increases glutathione production. Further, NAC is a direct free-radical scavenger and adds its protective effects to glutathione, further reducing oxidative damage in the brain.[87]

In a study comparing connective tissue (fibroblasts) of AD patients to controls, researchers found that NAC and lipoic acid supplements exerted an antioxidant protective effect, reducing oxidative damage and markers of cell death. NAC not only increased glutathione but also stabilized mitochondria. Mitochondria are the organelles inside cells that produce energy. Under inflammatory conditions they can become unstable and release damaging free radicals. NAC stabilizes the mitochondria and thereby reduces the oxidative damage in patients with AD.[88] Other research confirms the mitochondrial-stabilizing properties of NAC that reduce the production of oxidizing molecules and subsequently decrease programmed cell death.[89] Finally, in animal models of AD, NAC has been shown to delay age-associated memory impairments.[90]

Recommendations: First check with your doctor, then take a daily supplement of NAC, 500–1,500 mg per day.

Vitamin B$_{12}$, Folic Acid, and Homocysteine

It has been known for decades that vitamin B$_{12}$ and folic acid (vitamin B$_9$) are essential nutrients required for brain and body health. Deficiencies in these nutrients contribute to anemia[91] and psychiatric and neurological disorders,[92] including neural tube defects (spina bifida) in newborns.[93] More recent research has demonstrated that

215

these two vitamins also play a key role in cardiovascular health; deficiencies increase the risk of atherosclerosis, heart attacks, and strokes.[94] It has been well documented that chronic, high alcohol consumption depletes these vitamins as well as thiamine (vitamin B_1) and contributes to memory and language problems.[95] Other research has implicated deficiencies in these two vitamins with increased risk of AD.[96]

Deficiencies in vitamin B_{12} and folic acid contribute to a wide range of health problems because they are utilized in numerous physiological activities and metabolic processes in our bodies. These vitamins are required as cofactors for the production of the building blocks of our DNA (purine and thymidine),[97] production of neurotransmitters,[98] maintenance of brain cell health, production of blood by the bone marrow, and cell reproduction. One additional role both B_{12} and folic acid play in our bodies is to neutralize, recycle, and/or remove an inflammatory by-product of metabolism—homocysteine.

One pathway by which vitamin B_{12} and folic acid deficiencies contribute to increased risk for atherosclerosis, cognitive decline, and increased risk of AD is by the subsequent high levels of homocysteine.[99] Additionally, studies indicate that low levels of these essential B vitamins can accelerate brain volume loss. In a five-year study of 107 older adults (ages sixty-one to eighty-seven) living in the community (not in nursing homes), brain volume loss was greatest among those with the lowest B_{12} levels.[100] This is particularly concerning because studies have found that vitamin B_{12} deficiency occurs in more than one in five older adults but is often unrecognized because the symptoms are so subtle. Causes for this include impaired absorption (>60 percent of all cases), pernicious anemia (15–20 percent of all cases), and diets deficient in B_{12}.[101] Recently, studies have found that older adults with anemia are at higher risk of developing dementia than older adults without anemia.[102] The researchers could not determine the exact reason for this association between anemia and dementia, but possible factors include reduced oxygenation of the brain and overall increased oxidative stress, which affect both bone marrow and the brain, among other factors. Perhaps one other common link could be vitamin B deficiencies.

It is known that the low pH acidic environment of the stomach is necessary to activate the enzyme pepsinogen to become pepsin to release vitamin B_{12} from B_{12}-containing foods so that it can be absorbed. This has led some to hypothesize that recent medicines to treat heartburn (proton pump inhibitors [PPIs], Nexium [esomeprazole], Protonix [pantoprazole], Prilosec [omeprazole], Prevacid [lanzoprazole], etc.) have become so effective in raising stomach pH that they might be contributing to B_{12} deficiencies. In fact, some short-term studies found that use of these acid-reducing medicines did reduce B_{12} absorption.[103] However, multiple long-term studies have demonstrated that use of PPIs does not cause B_{12} deficiencies,[104] with the possible exception of two special situations. These are, first, in persons with a specific disorder in which tumors grow in the gastrointestinal system (Zollinger-Ellison syndrome)[105] and, second, in older adults who have reflux due to a stomach infection (*H. Pylori*) and develop chronic inflammation of the lining of the stomach (atrophic gastritis).[106] In these two circumstances, PPI use has been shown to reduce B_{12} absorption.

An additional problem for our health is that multiple gene mutations exist within the genes that metabolize and utilize folic acid and B_{12}. One of the most publicized is the *MTHFR* gene, which is involved in folic acid metabolism. It is well documented that persons with this gene defect cannot utilize folic acid properly and therefore have higher levels of the inflammatory by-product homocysteine.[107] Various studies have found this gene defect in 50–60 percent of individuals suffering with either coronary artery disease or depression.[108]

The good news is that as complex as all this seems, the solution is very simple: regular supplements of vitamin B_{12} and folic acid. If there is a history of depression or heart disease in either yourself or your family, I would recommend talking with your physician about getting genetic testing to determine if you have the *MTHFR* gene defect. If you do, simply taking the methylated form of folic acid, which is available in various strengths either over the counter or as a prescription, resolves the risk caused by the gene defect. And studies show that supplemental B vitamins do reduce the risk of AD.[109]

Recommendation: Talk with your doctor to determine your risk of deficiency and which supplemental form would be best for you.

Rhodiola Rosea

Rhodiola rosea, commonly known as golden root or rose root, is a perennial flowering plant in the Crassulaceae family that grows naturally in the arctic regions of Europe, Asia, and North America. It has been used in folk medicine for centuries to promote physical endurance and long life. The roots have a high concentration of phytochemicals such as flavonoids, monoterpenes, triterpenes, and phenols, which are pharmacologically active antioxidants, anti-inflammatories, anticancer, cardioprotective, and beneficial in the treatment of depression,[110] fatigue, and cognitive dysfunction.[111] Its strong neuroprotective effects have been documented in multiple studies.[112]

Because of the plethora of health-promoting benefits believed to be associated with this herb, a double-blind, placebo-controlled study evaluating the impact of *Rhodiola rosea* in treating individuals suffering from stress-related fatigue was conducted. Males and females between twenty and fifty-five years of age with diagnosis of chronic fatigue syndrome were selected. They were randomized into two groups, and for twenty-eight days one received 576 mg per day of *Rhodiola rosea* extract and the other received a placebo. The participants were evaluated on multiple scales: quality of life (SF-36 questionnaire), symptoms of fatigue

(Pines' burnout scale), depression (Montgomery-Asberg depression rating scale [MADRS]), attention (Conners' computerized continuous performance test II [CPT II]), and saliva cortisol response to awakening.

While both groups showed improvement in quality of life, depression, and burnout, significant positive effects were noted in the active-treatment group in the burnout and attention measures. The researchers concluded that "repeated administration of *R. rosea* extract SHR-5 exerts an anti-fatigue effect that increases mental performance, particularly the ability to concentrate, and decreases cortisol response to awakening stress in burnout patients with fatigue syndrome."[113]

More importantly for our study, *Rhodiola rosea* has demonstrated antiaging,[114] neuroprotective, and cognitive-enhancing properties. The cognitive-enhancing properties, such as improved attention, speed in task completion, and reduction in error rate, were seen within two hours of ingestion.[115] While the neuroprotective effects are likely related to the actions of the numerous phytochemicals, the cognitive improvement is most likely due to enhancement of neural-signaling chemicals such as dopamine and acetylcholine.[116]

Recommendation: Talk with your doctor about adding a daily morning dose of 150–600 mg of *Rhodiola rosea*.

Hormone Replacement Therapy

Over the last several decades there has been conflicting information regarding the potential benefit of hormone replacement therapy (HRT) for women. Initially, reports came out that HRT reduced heart disease risk in postmenopausal women. Later reports seemed to question the overall health benefits. One possible reason for this conflicting data may be the timing of when HRT is initiated. A recent report in the journal *Neurology* examining the results of a twenty-year follow-up study of over eight thousand Finnish women found that any estrogen replacement reduced the risk of AD; however, it did not reach statistical significance unless taken for ten years or more. For those who did take estrogen replacement for ten years or more, their risk of developing AD was significantly reduced by 40–50 percent.[117] This outcome was consistent with another study conducted in one county in Utah. In the Cache County, Utah, study investigators found that if estrogen was started within five years of menopause and continued for ten years or more, HRT was associated with reduction in developing AD.[118]

The timing or "critical window" theory may be one reason for conflicting data in studies that found no improved outcomes with HRT when the initiation of HRT happened after the first five years after menopause. This idea of a critical window is supported by other research that has demonstrated cardiovascular benefits to HRT if started within the first five years after menopause.[119]

Recommendation: Take this research to your doctor and discuss the risk versus benefits to you of starting HRT.

▪ LEARNING POINTS ▪

1. Omega-3 fatty acids (EPA/DHA) are essential to brain health, and individuals with high concentrations of these fats have less risk of AD.

2. There is no evidence that taking ginkgo biloba is of benefit in the prevention of AD, but there is some evidence that it improves memory and cognition in those who already have impairments.

3. Both high and low levels of vitamin D increase the risk of early death and dementia. Evidence supports an optimal blood level of 75–100 nmol/L.

4. Curcumin reduces *b*-amyloid in the brain and has anti-inflammatory benefits, but it is poorly absorbed without black pepper.

5. Walnuts reduce *b*-amyloid and the risk of dementia.

6. Green tea enhances cognition and memory and reduces *b*-amyloid buildup in the brain.

7. Pomegranate juice is rich in anti-inflammatory factors and reduces *b*-amyloid buildup in the brain, reducing risk of AD.

8. There is strong evidence that daily, mild-to-moderate (one to six cups) caffeinated coffee consumption reduces the risk of developing AD. Risks include increased possibility of seizure, sleep impairments, and reduced circulation.

9. Artificial sweeteners used in coffee are associated with increased risk of psychiatric decline; sugar and honey are not.

10. Vitamins E and C are antioxidants and reduce risk of AD; however, vitamin E should be obtained only from food. Vitamin C may be obtained from either food or supplements.

11. NAC is an antioxidant free-radical scavenger that stabilizes mitochondria; daily supplements are associated with a range of benefits, including reduced risk of AD.

12. Vitamin B_{12} and folic acid are essential vitamins that when deficient increase the risk of dementia. A subset of people has a gene defect that impairs their ability to absorb folic acid.

13. *Rhodiola rosea* is an herb with multiple physiologically active compounds with evidence that it slows aging, improves energy, and enhances cognition.

14. Estrogen (HRT), if started within five years of menopause, is associated with a reduction in AD risk, in one study as great as 40–50 percent.

▪ ACTION PLAN: THINGS TO DO ▪

1. Eat oily fish regularly (wild salmon, mackerel, sardines) or take omega-3 fatty acids supplements. The strongest evidence supports eating fish regularly.

2. Ask your doctor to test your vitamin D level and discuss options to achieve a blood level of 75–100 nmol/L.

3. Use curcumin in conjunction with black pepper, either in food preparation or as a daily supplement.

4. Eat a handful of raw walnuts daily.

5. Consider regular green tea consumption.

6. Drink one eight-ounce glass of 100 percent pomegranate juice daily.

7. Consult with your doctor about the potential risks versus benefits of drinking caffeinated coffee on a daily basis. Risks include increased possibility of seizure, sleep impairments, and reduced circulation.

8. Avoid artificial sweeteners completely in all foods and drinks.

9. Obtain vitamin E from food only (foods with the highest-to-lowest concentration of vitamin E include sunflower seeds, almonds, spinach, safflower oil, pumpkin, red pepper, asparagus, collard greens, and peanut butter). Vitamin C may be obtained from either food (citrus) or supplements.

10. Take a daily supplement of NAC; discuss dosing with your doctor.

11. Ask your doctor if your homocysteine, B_{12}, and folate levels should be checked and if you should be checked for the *MTHFR* gene defect. Take supplements as directed by your doctor once the testing is done.

12. Take a *Rhodiola rosea* supplement, 150–600 mg per day.

13. Talk with your doctor about estrogen replacement (HRT). (There is a lot of mixed information in the medical community about this so you might need to get the journal reference and take it with you.) Remember, the evidence suggests that if started within five years of menopause, HRT is associated with a reduction in AD risk.

16

Risk Factors for Dementia and How to Reduce the Risk

An ounce of prevention is worth a pound of cure.

Benjamin Franklin, in a letter to the
Pennsylvania Gazette, February 4, 1735

Aging—the slow decline in vitality and ability—is impacted by the choices we make in life. As we have seen throughout this book, any factor that increases inflammation and oxidative stress accelerates aging, while actions that are anti-inflammatory slow aging. In this chapter we will examine specific risk factors for developing Alzheimer's disease and specific actions that can be taken to minimize the risk and prevent the development of dementia. Some of the interventions are applicable to more than one risk factor.

ApoE4 Gene

Having two copies of this gene increases the risk of developing AD by 30–60 percent; however, this gene alone is not sufficient to cause AD. Those who apply the healthy choices listed in this book can reduce their risk and avoid developing AD—even if they have two copies of this gene.
Reduce risk by

- Regular exercise
- Mediterranean or vegan diet
- Avoiding use of substances that increase inflammation (tobacco, illegal drugs, excessive alcohol)
- Healthy spirituality and stress management
- Mental stimulation
- Getting 7–8 hours of sleep each night
- Drinking eight ounces of pomegranate juice daily
- Eating a handful of walnuts daily
- Getting adequate omega-3 fatty acids through either diet or supplements
- Having vitamin D level checked and keeping level at 75–100 nmol/L
- Ensuring adequate vitamin B_{12} and folic acid
- Getting vitamin E from food and daily vitamin C from food or supplements
- Using curcumin with black pepper regularly in food
- Daily NAC supplement
- Considering green tea and caffeinated coffee (balance this choice with risks of using these products)
- Avoiding artificial sweeteners
- Avoiding soft drinks

Oxidative Stress

Oxidation is the damage done to body tissues by molecules containing reactive oxygen capable of interacting and causing damage. Reduce risk by

- Avoiding oxidizing substances (illegal drugs, tobacco, heavy alcohol use) and minimizing charred, grilled, or fried foods (these cooking methods create advanced glycation endproducts, which are highly oxidizing)
- Exercising regularly (produces antioxidant cytokines that scavenge inflammatory cytokines)
- Regularly ingesting oily fish that is high in omega-3 fatty acids, which concentrates in neuronal membranes and scavenges free radicals, or taking supplements
- Eating fresh foods with color (berries, spinach, kale, etc.); flavonoids are antioxidant and scavenge free radicals
- Drinking eight ounces of pomegranate juice daily
- Eating walnuts (an antioxidant) daily
- Eating almonds, which are high in vitamin E that concentrates in neuronal membranes and scavenges free radicals
- Taking vitamin C supplements, which concentrate in cytoplasm (fluid inside neurons), scavenging free radicals and reactivating vitamin E
- Maintaining vitamin D level at 75–100 nmol/L
- Taking N-acetyl cysteine supplements, which stabilize mitochondria and reduce oxidative stress
- Using curcumin in diet, an anti-inflammatory that binds amyloid and helps clear it from the brain, reducing oxidative stress
- Avoiding fast foods and junk foods
- Avoiding artificial sweeteners

- Avoiding all soft drinks
- Coming into regular contact with the earth—your skin touching the earth (e.g., walk barefoot in the grass, swim in the ocean) in places where normal electrical conduction can occur to restore electron balance

Alcohol Abuse, Illegal Drugs, and Tobacco

Substance abuse is neurotoxic and oxidizing and interferes with the body's antioxidant enzymes, thereby accelerating aging and increasing the risk of dementia.

Reduce risk by

- Avoiding all tobacco and illegal drugs (see addendum for smoking-cessation action plan)
- Avoiding alcohol use; if use then do so moderately, never to drunkenness as intoxication is oxidizing; also, using only wine as distilled spirits are oxidizing
- Obtaining professional help if not able to achieve these goals

Sedentary Lifestyle

A sedentary lifestyle increases risk of obesity, which increases oxidative stress, denies the brain various neurotrophins (proteins that keep the neurons healthy and trigger new neuronal growth), increases inflammation and reduces anti-inflammatory factors produced with exercise, and increases insulin resistance.

Reduce risk by

- Regular exercise; consult your doctor before starting an exercise routine

- Starting low and going slow to avoid injury
- See specific recommendations at the end of chapter 8

Head Injury

The most common causes of head injuries are motor vehicle accidents, falls, and firearms, but other causes include contact sports, bicycle accidents, and assaults.

Reduce risk by

- Avoiding known risks such as boxing and extreme sports; if you participate, use head protection
- Wearing a helmet when bike riding
- Using seat belts, airbags, and antilock breaks
- Ensuring home environment is free of trip hazards

Diabetes Mellitus Type 2 (T2DM)/Glucose Intolerance

Type 2 diabetes doubles the risk of AD as anything that increases inflammation increases the risk of T2DM.

Reduce risk by

- Exercising regularly, which reduces inflammation and improves insulin sensitivity in addition to burning calories
- Eating an anti-inflammatory diet—Mediterranean or vegan
- Avoiding added sugars, particularly soft drinks, and eating fewer processed foods
- Avoiding junk food and fast foods
- Avoiding third-shift work and maintaining regular sleep; if you suspect obstructive sleep apnea, speak with your doctor about a sleep study

- Consulting your physician to discuss risk for T2DM and specific interventions to reduce risk

Obesity

Obesity is an inflammatory state that increases the risk of dementia and early death.

Reduce risk by

- Eating an anti-inflammatory diet—Mediterranean or vegan
- Exercising regularly—walk twenty minutes each day; when combined with a vegan or Mediterranean diet, the impact is even more robust; both improve insulin sensitivity, leading to greater fat burning by the body
- Addressing known risk factors such as sleep apnea and medical conditions (hypothyroid, etc.)
- Reducing mental stress
- Sleeping eight hours each night
- Fasting twelve hours between dinner and breakfast each day
- Changing diet to alter gut flora (see chap. 5)
- Considering professional help and working with your physician if these measures do not work

Western Diet

The Western diet is an inflammatory diet high in processed foods, sugars, trans fats, advanced glycation end-products, and dairy, all of which increase the risk of dementia.

Reduce risk by

- Changing to vegan or Mediterranean diet
- Limiting added sugar

- Eating regular servings of fish
- Reducing dairy products; milk and cheese are inflammatory
- Avoiding all soft drinks
- Avoiding artificial sweeteners
- Avoiding junk food and fast foods
- Regularly eating fruit, walnuts, and almonds

High Blood Pressure

High blood pressure increases the risk of both vascular and Alzheimer's dementias. Reduce risk by

- Seeing your physician for treatment; studies show that controlling high blood pressure reduces risk for dementia[1]

Low Cognitive Stimulation

If you don't use it, you lose it—the law of exertion. If you want to keep your mental acuity, then you must use your mental abilities regularly. Failure to do so accelerates cognitive and mental decline. Reduce risk by

- Staying mentally active
- Doing puzzles
- Taking art lessons
- Learning to play an instrument
- Teaching a class at church, a neighborhood association, or other community group
- Learning a new language
- Taking a class at a community college

- Participating in a Bible study
- Taking dance lessons

Depression

Depression increases the risk of dementia.[2]

Reduce risk by

- Effective depression treatment
- Consulting your physician
- Recommendations listed in this book for reducing the risk of dementia in regard to exercise, diet, stress management, sleep, avoidance of toxins, and so on

Social Isolation

Loneliness and social isolation cause increased stress, resulting in increased activation of inflammatory cascades, and are associated with increased risk of dementia.

Reduce risk by

- Joining a group with shared interests—for example, a religious group such as a church, synagogue, or mosque, or a book club, an exercise group, a community outreach agency, or a golf club
- Starting a group in an activity you enjoy and inviting others to join you
- Volunteering at a local hospital, Goodwill, animal shelter, soup kitchen, or any other such program—helping others not only improves social connectedness but also activates the love circuits of the brain and calms the fear circuits, thereby reducing inflammatory cascades and slowing the aging process

Psychological Stress

Unresolved mental stress activates the brain's alarm circuitry, which activates the immune system, increasing inflammation and contributing to oxidative stress, higher rates of metabolic syndrome, depression, and increased risk of dementia.

Reduce risk by

- Forgiving those who have done you wrong
- Practicing healthy spirituality with regular meditation on a God of love
- Taking a weekly vacation in time to set aside the routine stresses of life
- Spending time in natural settings
- Resolving existential anxiety such as fear about death and dying
- Considering seeing a counselor if you find yourself constantly stressed, worried, anxious, or ruminating on negative and pessimistic thoughts

Chronic Sleep Deprivation

Approximately one in three Americans is chronically sleep deprived, sleeping fewer than seven hours per night. Sleep is one of four physical requirements for life, along with air, water, and food. Chronic sleep deprivation is devastating to brain health. Without regular adequate sleep brain function is impaired, particularly the part of the brain in which we attend, focus, organize, plan, self-restrain, self-calm, and modulate mood.

Reduce risk by

- Establishing a stable sleep routine with structured and enforced going-to-bed and getting-out-of bed times to ensure 7–8 hours of sleep each night

- Sleeping at night and avoiding third-shift work, if possible; sleeping in harmony with normal biorhythms, meaning sleep at night and not during the day; third-shift workers, even if sleeping eight hours every twenty-four hours, still have a higher risk of obesity, mental health problems, dementia, and early death than those who sleep at night
- Sleeping in a dark room and taking actions to avoid environmental disruptions (keep animals out of room, use sound machine to minimize arousing noises, keep room cool, etc.)
- Avoiding eating late at night
- Considering getting a sleep study if chronically fatigued, a heavy snorer, obese, or have chronic headaches as these are symptoms of obstructive sleep apnea

One additional recommendation to reduce risk of dementia is to drink adequate amounts of water to maintain good hydration. Water is the single largest component of our bodies, comprising well over half of our body weight. Every cell of the body requires water. Water is essential for the functioning of our cells and the removal of waste products of metabolism. Dehydration shrinks the cells of the body, and their function becomes impaired. This results in increased oxidative stress and inability to clear toxins, which result in greater damage to our cells, including our brains. Concentration, memory, and general alertness can be negatively affected by dehydration. An average adult should drink eight, eight-ounce glasses of water each day, and more if exercising vigorously or working in hot, humid environments.

▪ LEARNING POINTS ▪

1. There are known risks to developing dementia—some inherited, others lifestyle related.

2. The inherited risks can be effectively reduced by healthy life-style choices so that AD can be prevented.

3. While we can't avoid aging, we can make choices that slow the decline in abilities; maintain vitality, autonomy, and in-dependence; and prevent the development of dementia.

17

Caring for a Loved One with Dementia

I look into your face,
Your eyes stare into space,
I try to search deep into your soul,
To find the man I once knew,
But he is not there.
The emptiness goes beyond compare.
Where are you . . . ? I ask.
Where have you gone . . . ?

Carolyn A. Haynali, "The Empty Face,"
Poetry from the Heart by
an Alzheimer's Caregiver, 2005

Her freckled face, strawberry blonde hair, and petite stature made me smile when I first saw her. Despite her middle age, she projected a youthful aura. She initially reminded me of a high-school cheerleader, until I saw the first glimpse of the pain she worked so hard to conceal, the heartache that was eclipsing the light from her eyes.

Margaret was forty-four years old and for the last five years had been the primary caregiver to her mother, who was slowly dying from Alzheimer's disease. Initially, it wasn't so bad. Mom could still do all the routine things such as bathe, toilet herself, dress herself, and prepare meals. In the beginning Margaret only supervised her medications and finances. At first she didn't really notice much was wrong. There was the occasional forgotten conversation, misplaced item, and inability to recall a name, place, or date, but her mother always knew her and was glad to see her. But that was five years ago.

The neuronal grim reaper had taken many victims since then. Mom's brain was now much smaller than it once had been. With each passing day, with each brain cell lost, a little more of Mom faded away until all that remained was a living, empty shell that little resembled the person her mom used to be.

Margaret's mother could no longer dress herself, feed herself, or bathe or toilet herself. It had been several years since she had known the time, date, or where she was. It was only the rare occasion that Mother recognized Margaret, and more often than not she referred to her daughter as "mama." Mom would frequently wander through the house at night, see people who didn't exist, and accuse Margaret of being an intruder. Margaret couldn't remember the last time she had a full night's sleep, and she spent all day and most of every night caring for her parent. She was tired. But physical fatigue was not why she had come to see me.

Margaret had come to me because she felt torn, trapped, and consumed with guilt. Her mother had made her promise some years before that Margaret would never put her into a nursing home. This promise was made before either of them knew about the Alzheimer's. Margaret had worked exhaustively to keep that promise but was wearing out. She physically could no longer keep up. She needed help and thought more frequently of placing her mother in a nursing home, but with every such thought she was pummeled with guilt: *How could I just abandon my mother after all she did for me? A loving daughter wouldn't do such a thing. You promised Mom you wouldn't.*

Margaret's internal struggle is a common battle faced by those caring for a parent who is unable to care for themselves. Often people find themselves in a terrible bind between what their heart would prefer to do and what in reality they are capable of doing. For many, rather than choosing what is objectively best they instead push on with what they would prefer, until they exhaust themselves so severely that they collapse and can no longer function. Only then do they get the help they have needed for quite some time. This seems to be especially true when dealing with parents who are aging.

I asked Margaret, If her mother had a broken leg, would she try to set the bone herself or seek professional help? If her mother needed heart surgery, would she clear off the kitchen table and do it herself or get a heart surgeon? Because her mother's decline was so gradual, so insidious, so slow, she never really stopped to define the objective medical criteria that would necessitate seeking external help. The question Margaret needed to answer was, Did her mother have a condition that objectively required assistance beyond that which Margaret could reasonably provide? In fact, would Margaret, by refusing to get such assistance, be placing her mother in greater danger?

The answer was obviously yes. Mother had wandered out of the house one night after Margaret fell into an exhausted sleep. Neighbors, several blocks away, called the police when Mom tried to get into their house screaming nonsense. Margaret realized that in order to fulfill her loving obligation to Mom, she needed to find assistance in caring for her.

At long last, Mom was placed in a very nice nursing facility that specialized in treating those with dementia. She was receiving more comprehensive care than Margaret could give, but Margaret didn't significantly improve. She continued to be stressed, conflicted, torn, and guilt ridden. There was more troubling her than she had yet disclosed.

After gentle prodding she finally told me the dark secret that had been troubling her, the shameful thoughts that had been eating at her, the awful ideas that had stolen her peace. Margaret broke into tears and said, "For the last year I have wished my mother would just die. How horrible is that? How could I? What kind of a daughter would have thoughts wishing her mother would die?"

I sat quietly for a few moments, allowing the words she had spoken to sink in. Then I said, "Margaret, let's say I had two buttons on the wall. If you push the button on the left your mother will be miraculously and instantly healed, restored to vitality, her mind and health fully recovered, and she will be as you had always known her. If you push the button on the right your mother will instantly die. Now, which button would you push?"

"The one on the left!" she said instantly.

"Margaret, you have never wanted your mother to die. You have only wanted her suffering to stop. You realize when she dies her suffering will be over. But you would restore her to health if you could. Isn't that right?"

Margaret paused, eyes wide in contemplation, then sobbed as she nodded her head, overcome with relief. Margaret's situation is representative of the struggles many people face and many more will soon face when caring for aging parents: the objective needs of their condition, which require time, money, energy, in addition to the subjective struggles of love, grief, guilt, frustration, and anger. One often is torn between competing responsibilities, those to one's own children, grandchildren, and spouse versus those to aging parents. Should I keep Mother in the home, impacting my family, missing their events in order to care for a parent? What is the cost to the rest of the family? Should I put my parent in a long-term care facility? Is that right after all they have done for me? This is often the struggle.

There are many websites with helpful and practical advice as well as resources to assist in caring for a loved one with dementia. Following is a list of a few of them:

- National Institute on Aging: Alzheimer's Caregiving (www.nia.nih.gov/health/alzheimers/caregiving)
- Alzheimer's Association: Caregiver Center (www.alz.org/care/overview.asp)
- WebMD: Alzheimer's Disease Care (www.webmd.com/alzheimers/daily-care-alzheimers)

These sites are filled with practical guidance and are readily accessible; therefore, I am not going to reproduce all that information here. My goal in this section is to facilitate honesty, to help people acknowledge that these struggles are real and to bring them out in the open so they can be resolved. Only then can these real-life dilemmas be evaluated and addressed effectively.

We must also recognize that every situation is unique and what works best for one family might not be the best solution for another. I will describe several principles that guide our decisions, but the situation will determine the specific action that is best.

For instance, love—seeking to do what is best for the other—is a principle, but the situation determines what action love takes. Do you let your parent drive or do you take the keys? Love wants a parent to have as much autonomy as possible but at the same time wants to protect them from serious risk of injuring themselves or others. What determines whether the keys to the car are taken or not? *The actual functional ability of the parent.* When dealing with our aging parents, the principle of love leads us to seek what is best for them, but the situation will determine what action is actually needed.

Can you identify the principle at work in the famous adage "Love your neighbor as yourself"? I learned this principle when running an inpatient psychiatric unit. The first rule of a psychiatric unit is staff safety—not patient safety. Why? Because if the staff are not safe, then the patients are not safe and no care is provided. This principle is true for everyone who helps others. A farmer who won't eat will not feed anyone. In order to be of use, to be capable of helping others, we must take actions necessary to safeguard, protect, and promote our own health. If we don't, then instead of being in a position to help others we will need to be cared for by others. Even Jesus Christ regularly took time away from the needy masses to rest, eat, and spend time in prayer in order to rejuvenate himself for ministry to the people.

Caretakers need to establish the minimum objective requirements they must meet in order to maintain their own health, energy, and wellness, including mental well-being, so that they avoid exhaustion, burnout, and physical and mental breakdown. This would include such things as a healthy diet, routine exercise, and regular sleep but also time away from caregiving for mental decompression and rejuvenation. Failure to attend to one's own health will result in wearing out; rather than being able to provide care to another, the caregiver breaks down and will need to be cared for by others.

With this in mind, let's review some practical approaches to caring for an aging parent with Alzheimer's disease.

Be sure your parent has a health-care provider who is familiar with the unique health problems of aging and specifically with dementia. This may entail having a primary care physician as well as a specialist such as a neurologist or psychiatrist to manage the dementia-related problems.

In conjunction with your loved one's physician, set reasonable goals for your parent. These goals will change with time, but examples of reasonable goals for late-stage AD would be maintaining nightly sleep, good nutrition, avoiding hostility and anger outbursts, preventing wandering off, and stopping hallucinations.

Establish objective criteria that automatically trigger changes in care. For example, one reasonable goal would be to maintain regular sleep of seven to eight hours each night. A measurable criterion that would trigger a change in care would be a change in sleep. If your loved one is up wandering throughout the night unable to sleep, this should trigger a visit to the doctor, who will assess if something has changed in their underlying health—such as a urinary tract infection. If such a problem is identified and treated and sleep is stabilized, then care at home continues. However, if the inability to maintain regular nightly sleep despite medical intervention occurs, this would be an example of a measurable criterion that for some families would be the trigger to seek placement in a long-term care facility.

Establishing such criteria before they occur can make the process of executing the action (moving a loved one into long-term care) easier. It would be understood that this is based on the needs of the aging loved one. It's not an *unwillingness* to provide care but an actual *inability* to provide the care needed.

Safety at Home

Many of the actions one needs to take when dealing with loved ones suffering with dementia are similar to dealing with small children—making the home safe. When the memory of a person with AD is impaired they may start activities and then get distracted and forget what they started, contributing to dangerous situations. For instance, a person might start cooking or ironing, and then the phone rings or a deer walks by a window and they walk over to look, and so on. But having left the stove or iron, they forget what they were doing and don't turn it off, thus creating a potential fire hazard. When persons who are at home have this level of memory impairment it is important to protect them and everyone else from such dangers. One way to do this is to put the iron away where it cannot be accessed and turn the electrical breaker or gas off to the stove or range so it cannot be turned on. Matches, lighters, and other fire starters should be removed, guns should be locked away, and medicines should be placed in locked and secured containers. Medications should not only be locked up but also be dispensed by a third party as people with dementia often either forget to take their meds or forget they have already taken them and take multiple doses.

Other actions to promote safety include changing out shoes with shoelaces for ones with Velcro straps. These are not only easier for the aging person to manage on their own but also reduce tripping and falling risks. Ensure that shoes are worn most of the time, even indoors, to reduce risk of foot injury. Circulation is often compromised in the elderly and frequently there is neuropathy, the loss of temperature and pain sensation, which means an elderly person can injure their foot and not know it. If this happens infection can set in and cause serious problems, especially in diabetics.

If your loved one has a real risk of getting up and wandering at night, consider a bed alarm, which will sound should they get out of bed. This can allow you to sleep without worrying about whether your loved one is still in bed.

Guardianship versus Power of Attorney

I am not an attorney and am not giving legal advice, but I am pointing out some circumstances that call for legal counsel. One of these is determining legal authority—power of attorney or guardianship. The difference between guardianship and power of attorney (POA) is that POA is *granted by a person* who is competent and who authorizes another person to act for them in legal matters. In this case, it would be granted by the parent to the child. Granting power of attorney to someone else does not remove the ability of the person who granted the POA to act on their own behalf. Further, POA can be rescinded by the one granting it at any time.

This means if your parent has granted you POA you have legal authorization to act for them in any matter for which the power was granted you (sometimes the POA is limited to specific actions such as medical decision-making; other times it is a general POA). However, your parent can still legally take actions for themselves. Guardianship, on the other hand, is granted by a court and is given when a person is no longer capable of acting in their own behalf. Guardianship removes the legal right of a person to act in their own behalf in legal matters, which means your parent cannot sell their house, open a credit card, buy a car, write checks, donate money, and so on without the authorization of the guardian. This is an important distinction to understand, as there are less-than-honorable people in our society who prey upon the elderly. Obtaining guardianship, when it is appropriate, is one way to protect our parents from such exploitation.

Avoid Arguing

When dealing with a parent who is no longer reasoning at their previous level, who forgets, who may draw erroneous conclusions, who may even misidentify loved ones and believe they are in a different time and place, it is important not to argue with them or seek to make them admit they are wrong. It is also important not to get your feelings hurt or take accusations personally. Arguing and demanding your parent admit he or she is wrong will only cause agitation and hostility and will not result in learning. Remember, your parent has lost the brain matter necessary to learn and remember so arguing with them is pointless.

As individuals dement, their capacity to assimilate and process new information is strained, and life can become overwhelming and stressful. Such things as meeting new people, navigating the parking lot, processing the sights and noises from people in a store can be frightening and distressful. Commonly, as people begin to lose cognitive abilities, they will choose to isolate and stay at home where things are routine and familiar. If this happens do not force your parent to attend activities that are stressful to them; instead, consider ways to minimize the amount of mental tracking and strain that will be placed on them. In this way the activities will be less stressful and they will be more likely to engage.

Because a person who is deteriorating has impaired ability to assimilate and learn new information, including new surroundings, if your loved one has to be moved to a long-term care facility do everything possible to make their new abode feel homey and familiar. Bring pictures, furniture, blankets, beds, towels, and anything that can be reasonably incorporated into the new facility with them. This reduces their feeling of strangeness and brings comfort, reducing agitation and acting out.

Finally, don't go it alone. If you have supportive family, reach out and get help. If you don't have family, then reach out to your church, neighbors, or local Alzheimer's Association. Connecting with others provides encouragement, understanding, and real help in carrying out the caregiving responsibilities.

As long as we are living, we cannot avoid growing older—the only question is how do we want our passages through time to unfold? I hope this book has inspired you not only to live long but also to live well and to incorporate into your life these various evidenced-based practices, which not only promote health but actually slow decline, preserve function, and prevent dementia.

▪ LEARNING POINTS ▪

1. Caring for an aging parent is a time of great emotional anguish filled with conflicting feelings and additional responsibilities.

2. In order to be able to provide care to another we must be vigilant to maintain our own health. This requires thoughtful establishment of those things necessary for our own self-care.

3. Ensure your parent is under the care of a physician familiar with the problems of the elderly and those with dementia.

4. Establish, in conjunction with the physician, a reasonable list of goals.

5. Take specific actions, as necessary, to make the home safe.

6. Establish measurable criteria that will automatically trigger a change in care.

7. If you must move your loved one to a new living situation, bring as many of their personal belongings as possible to make the new place familiar to them.

8. Determine and establish the best legal status for your situation—power of attorney or guardianship.

9. Don't argue when your parent doesn't remember things.

10. Don't take accusations personally.

11. Don't go it alone—get help.

Addendum

Dr. Jennings's Smoking-Cessation Strategy

I f you or someone you know is struggling to stop smoking, following are some simple steps that can help you or them break free from nicotine's grasp.

1. *Stop caffeine.* In the brain caffeine causes a neurobiologically increased craving for nicotine. Therefore, drinking caffeinated beverages increases the craving for cigarettes and makes it more difficult to quit smoking. If you have been drinking more than six caffeinated beverages per day, taper down by two drinks per day until off the caffeine. This taper will minimize caffeine-withdrawal headaches and fatigue. Plan to stop smoking after the caffeine has been eliminated. (Once you are cigarette free for a month, you can cautiously reintroduce one to two caffeinated beverages per day if you desire. However, be prepared to experience sudden nicotine cravings.)

2. *Avoid alcohol.* Alcohol causes a neurobiologically increased craving for nicotine, just as caffeine does, but alcohol also interferes with the functioning of the prefrontal cortex. This means it undermines judgment, resolve, and willpower, and the combined effects of increased cravings and diminished willpower typically lead to relapse of smoking. (If you are a social drinker you can reintroduce an occasional alcoholic beverage once you are tobacco free for one month, but be prepared for the potential onset of nicotine cravings.)

3. *Set a date.* Set a date for your last cigarette and stick to it. When the date comes, get rid of all your cigarettes, ashtrays, and smoking paraphernalia.

4. *Identify triggers and replace.* Smoking is not only a physical addiction; it is also a psychological one—a conditioned response. Smokers have certain habits or times in which they routinely smoke. These habits will trigger a craving for a cigarette. For instance, a smoker who has the habit of smoking when he gets into the car will experience a desire to smoke whenever he gets into the car. If the habit is smoking after a meal, then anticipate a craving for a cigarette after each meal, or after a shower, and so on. Sometimes triggers can be emotional such as smoking when angry or frustrated. Take an inventory of your habit patterns and recognize your triggers, and then either avoid them (if possible) or plan a replacement, such as popping a Tic Tac or chewing gum instead of smoking.

5. *Join forces.* If your spouse smokes and is willing to stop, then team up together and implement a smoking-cessation plan jointly. Encourage each other during this process. If your partner doesn't smoke, solicit their involvement as your coach and partner to encourage, praise, and support you during this time.

6. *Exercise.* Exercise not only improves cardiovascular health, resulting in improved lung function, but also results in the

production of brain chemicals (endorphins and enkephalins) that reduce cravings. If you haven't been exercising, start with easy exercises and go slowly to avoid injuries. Also, check with your primary care physician if you have any health problems that could preclude exercise.

7. *Take charge of your imagination.* Within a few hours of the last cigarette, a smoker will typically experience cravings. This is often the turning point in the battle to be free of smoking. If you are not prepared when the cravings hit, the desire will grab hold of you and you may begin to imagine things, such as the familiar sound of opening a pack, the feel of the flick of the lighter, the smell of the smoke, and the taste of the tobacco. Such imaginary events fuel greater cravings, undermine resolve, and typically result in a relapse into smoking. One way to avoid this is to be prepared to take purposeful charge of the imagination. When the cravings come, imagine pulling a flip-top box of cigarettes out, opening the top, and seeing cockroaches come crawling out on your hand, or imagine it is filled with maggots wiggling around. Use an imagery that will cause an emotion of revulsion and disgust.

Genuine victory over an addiction is not achieved by gaining more facts about the harm of the habit. Smokers don't need more education on cancer risks or heart disease risks. In order to be genuinely free, a smoker (or any addict) must experience a change in the way they feel about their addiction. When a smoker thinks of smoking, they usually experience some positive emotion, "yeah," "that's nice," or "oh that's good," what is commonly called a *warm fuzzy*. Warm fuzzies need to be replaced with emotions of revulsion. What emotion would you experience if someone offered you a fresh bowl of dog feces with a spoon? As the smell wafted up toward you, would you experience revulsion? If you had the same emotional response toward smoking, what would be the chances you would put one in your mouth? You have the power to imagine cigarettes in some way that engenders revulsion rather than a warm fuzzy. Do it!

8. *Drink plenty of water and fresh juices.* For the first week (at least), be sure to flush your system with plenty of water and fresh fruit juice as this will help remove toxins, free radicals, and other damaging products caused by smoking.

9. *Buddy up.* Solicit a close friend to be your buddy during the first week of the cessation process. If during this time a craving comes that seems more than you can handle, call your buddy to talk you through it. Tell your buddy why you need them and what their role is, and get their permission to call anytime day or night for that week. Cravings come in waves—if you resist, the craving will pass. The craving will return later but if resisted will pass again. Over the course of the first week cravings will get weaker and weaker until they remit for good. The physical withdrawal from nicotine lasts only a week; if you can make it past seven days, the physical portion will be over. It will then be a matter of changing habit patterns, thought processes, and feelings about the addiction.

10. *Pray.* Don't forget the power of prayer. Ask God into your heart and mind and obtain his strength each day. Be thoughtful toward him and call on him anytime throughout the day or night. Ask God to change your desires, strengthen your willpower, diminish the cravings, and enhance your mind's ability to think clearly. Ask friends and family to lift you up in prayer, especially during the first week, soliciting special intervention to help during this time. But remember, God will not send an angel from heaven to snatch the cigarette from your mouth. You must willfully choose to say no in order to receive God's power to succeed.

11. *Clean everything.* Clean car, rugs, clothes, curtains, windows—get the smell of tobacco out of your life and bring in a clean freshness to start your new healthy living.

12. *Avoid mental games.* Don't tell yourself, "I am going to quit—unless I have a really bad day" or "This is my last cigarette—unless I feel overwhelmed." Such thinking leaves an escape clause from total cessation, and most people will unconsciously create the necessary circumstances in which to exercise their secret escape clause. Be real with yourself. When you decide to quit tell yourself that it doesn't matter how bad it gets, you are not smoking again. No escape clauses!

13. *Remind yourself the reasons for quitting.* Make a list of all the benefits for quitting. This would include health, monetary savings, and no more hassles finding a place to smoke. But even more important, remind yourself of all the loved ones whom you will be benefiting. You will increase the likelihood of being there when your daughter graduates, your son gets married, your first grandchild is born, as well as no longer exposing your loved ones to secondhand smoke. Remind yourself of all the additional joy you will have in life. Write this list down, put it in your wallet, and when discouraged pull it out and look at it. Maybe put it near a picture of your spouse or child. They will be proud of you!

14. *Consider nicotine gum or patches.* Nicotine gum or patches should not be used if still smoking as both together could cause lethal doses of nicotine. Nicotine gum and patches continue to supply the brain with nicotine so the physical addiction will not be resolved until all sources of nicotine are removed. However, for some individuals the nicotine gum or patch allows them time to break the psychological triggers and smoking habit pattern, clean their house, and then taper off the gum or patch, finally quitting all of it. This is not necessary for everyone but does help many.

15. *Consider medications.* There are a variety of prescription medications available to assist with smoking cessation. Consult with your doctor to see if any of these might be helpful during this time. However, medications are not a substitute for all the steps above, and medications do not magically remove a smoking addiction. Medications can, for some persons, reduce the intensity of the physical cravings—that is all. They do not break habits, they do not change the imagination, they do not remove toxins from the body, and they do not instill a revulsion for tobacco. If medicine is used as an additional aid to stop smoking, the smoker will still be required to actively choose to put the cigarettes down, change habits, and implement all the steps above.

NOTES

Chapter 1 The Problem of Aging

1. Nadine R. Sahyoun et al., "Trends in Causes of Death among the Elderly," Centers for Disease Control and Prevention, March 2001, http://www.cdc.gov/nchs /data/ahcd/agingtrends/01death.pdf.

2. Sahyoun et al., "Trends in Causes of Death," http://www.cdc.gov/nchs/data /ahcd/agingtrends/01death.pdf.

3. Jean-Yves Fagon, "Acute respiratory failure in the elderly," *Critical Care* 10, no. 4 (July 25, 2006): 151, http://www.ncbi.nlm.nih.gov/pmc/articles/PMC 1751014/.

4. "Disability Characteristics," US Census Bureau, 2011, http://factfinder2 .census.gov/faces/tableservices/jsf/pages/productview.xhtml?pid=ACS_11_1YR _S1810&prodType=table.

Chapter 2 Developing a Healthy Brain

1. James R. Healey, "6 killed in GM cars with faulty ignition switches," *USA Today*, updated February 14, 2014, http://www.usatoday.com/story/money/cars /2014/02/13/gm-recall/5448319/.

2. Chang Hyung Hong et al., "Anemia and risk of dementia in older adults: findings from the Health ABC study," *Neurology* 81, no. 6 (August 6, 2013): 528–33.

3. G. Biessels et al., "Risk of dementia in diabetes mellitus: a systematic review," *Lancet Neurology* 5, no. 1 (January 2006): 64–74.

4. R. A. Whitmer et al., "Midlife cardiovascular risk factors and risk of dementia in late life," *Neurology* 64, no. 2 (January 25, 2005): 277–81.

5. Tatsuo Yamamoto et al., "Association between self-reported dental health status and onset of dementia: a 4-year prospective cohort study of older Japanese adults from the Aichi Gerontological Evaluation Study (AGES) Project," *Psychosomatic Medicine* 74, no. 3 (April 2012): 241–48, https://doi.org/10.1097 /PSY.0b013e318246dffb.

6. P. S. Stein et al., "Tooth loss, dementia and neuropathology in the Nun Study," *Journal of the American Dental Association* 138, no. 10 (October 2007): 1314–22.

7. Michael J. Proulx, "Bottom-up guidance in visual search for conjunctions," *Journal of Experimental Psychology: Human Perception and Performance* 33, no. 1 (February 2007): 48–56, https://doi.org/10.1037/0096-1523.33.1.48.

8. S. Jay Olshansky et al., "Differences in life expectancy due to race and educational differences are widening, and many may not catch up," *Health Affairs* 31, no. 8 (August 2012): 1803–13.

9. Kirk I. Erickson et al., "Exercise training increases size of hippocampus and improves memory," *Proceedings of the National Academy of Sciences of the United States of America* 108, no. 7 (February 2011): 3017–22, https://doi.org/10.1073/pnas.1015950108.

10. A. Danese et al., "Adverse childhood experiences and adult risk factors for age-related disease: depression, inflammation, and clustering of metabolic risk markers," *Archives of Pediatrics & Adolescent Medicine* 163, no. 12 (December 2009): 1135–43.

Chapter 3 Epigenetics and Aging

1. M. E. Pembrey et al., "Sex-specific, male-line transgenerational responses in humans," *European Journal of Human Genetics* 14, no. 2 (February 2006): 159–66, https://www.ncbi.nlm.nih.gov/pubmed/16391557.

2. Bastiaan T. Heijmans et al., "Persistent epigenetic differences associated with prenatal exposure to famine in humans," *Proceedings of the National Academy of Sciences of the United States of America* 105, no. 44 (November 2008): 17046–49, https://doi.org/10.1073/pnas.0806560105.

3. Alison K. Shae and Meir Steiner, "Cigarette smoking during pregnancy," *Nicotine & Tobacco Research* 10, no. 2 (February 1 2008): 267–78, https://doi.org/10.1080/14622200701825908; Stanley Zammit et al., "Maternal tobacco, cannabis and alcohol use during pregnancy and risk of adolescent psychotic symptoms in offspring," *British Journal of Psychiatry* 195, no. 4 (September 2009): 294–300, http://bjp.rcpsych.org/cgi/content/abstract/195/4/294.

4. Bonnie R. Joubert et al., "DNA methylation in newborns and maternal smoking in pregnancy: genome-wide consortium meta-analysis," *American Journal of Human Genetics* 98, no. 4 (April 2016): 680–96, http://www.cell.com/ajhg/fulltext/S0002-9297(16)00070-7.

5. Mina Rydell et al., "Prenatal exposure to tobacco and future nicotine dependence: population-based cohort study," *British Journal of Psychiatry* 200, no. 3 (March 2012): 202–9, https://doi.org/10.1192/bjp.bp.111.100123.

6. Michael S. Kobor and Joanne Weinberg, "FOCUS ON: Epigenetics and fetal alcohol spectrum disorders," National Institute on Alcohol Abuse and Alcoholism, *Alcohol Research & Health* 34, no. 1, http://pubs.niaaa.nih.gov/publications/arh341/29-37.htm.

7. Ruth Little et al., "Fetal growth and moderate drinking in early pregnancy," *American Journal of Epidemiology* 123, no. 2 (February 1986): 270–78; A. C. Huizink and E. J. Mulder, "Maternal smoking, drinking or cannabis use during

pregnancy and neurobehavioral and cognitive functioning in human offspring," *Neuroscience & Biobehavioral Reviews* 30, no. 1 (2006): 24–41; K. Sayal et al., "Prenatal alcohol exposure and gender differences in childhood mental health problems: a longitudinal population-based study," *Pediatrics* 119, no. 2 (February 2007).

8. Steven L. Youngentob and John I. Glendinning, "Fetal ethanol exposure increases ethanol intake by making it smell and taste better," *Proceedings of the National Academy of Sciences of the United States of America* 106, no. 13 (March 31, 2009): 5359–64.

9. Bradley S. Peterson et al., "Effects of prenatal exposure to air pollutants (polycyclic aromatic hydrocarbons) on the development of brain white matter, cognition, and behavior in later childhood," *Journal of the American Medical Association: Psychiatry* 72, no. 6 (June 2015): 531–40, https://doi.org/10.1001/jamapsychiatry.2015.57.

10. R. M. Pearson et al., "Association between maternal depressogenic cognitive style during pregnancy and offspring cognitive style 18 years later," *American Journal of Psychiatry* 170, no. 4 (April 2013): 434–41.

11. John J. Medina, "The epigenetics of stress," *Psychiatric Times* (April 7, 2010): 16.

12. "Salimbene: On Frederick II, 13th Century," *Medieval Sourcebook*, Fordham University, January 1996, http://legacy.fordham.edu/halsall/source/salimbene1.html.

13. I. C. Weaver et al., "Epigenetic programming by maternal behavior," *Nature Neuroscience* 7, no. 8 (August 2004): 847–54, http://www.ncbi.nlm.nih.gov/pubmed/15220929.

14. B. Labonté et al., "Genome-wide epigenetic regulation by early-life trauma," *Archives of General Psychiatry* 69, no. 7 (July 2012): 722–31.

15. A. Danese et al., "Adverse childhood experiences and adult risk factors for age-related disease: depression, inflammation, and clustering of metabolic risk markers," *Archives of Pediatrics & Adolescent Medicine* 63, no. 12 (December 2009): 1135–43.

16. J. Bick et al., "Childhood adversity and DNA methylation of genes involved in the hypothalamus-pituitary-adrenal axis and immune system: whole-genome and candidate-gene associations," *Development and Psychopathology* 24, no. 4 (November 2012): 1417–25. See also Judith E. Carroll et al., "Childhood abuse, parental warmth, and adult multisystem biological risk in the Coronary Artery Risk Development in Young Adults study," *Proceedings of the National Academy of Sciences of the United States of America* 110, no. 42 (October 15, 2013): 17149–53; M. Kelly-Irving et al., "Adverse childhood experiences and premature all-cause mortality," *European Journal of Epidemiology* 28, no. 9 (September 2013): 721–34; L. K. Gilbert et al., "Childhood adversity and adult chronic disease: an update from ten states and the District of Columbia, 2010," *American Journal of Preventive Medicine* 48, no. 3 (March 2015): 345–49.

17. E. Levy-Gigi et al., "Association among clinical response, hippocampal volume, and FKBP5 gene expression in individuals with posttraumatic stress disorder receiving cognitive behavioral therapy," *Biological Psychiatry* 74, no. 11 (December 2013): 793–800.

18. Kirsten Weir, "Forgiveness can improve mental and physical health: research shows how to get there," *Monitor on Psychology* 48, no. 1 (January 2017): 30.

19. Junko A. Arai et al., "Transgenerational rescue of a genetic defect in long-term potentiation and memory formation by juvenile enrichment," *Journal of Neuroscience* 29, no. 5 (February 2009): 1496–1502, https://doi.org/10.1523/JN EUROSCI.5057-08.2009.

Chapter 4 Our Genes and Aging

1. M. Egan et al., "The human genome: mutations," *American Journal of Psychiatry* 159, no. 1 (January 2002): 12.

2. "Prader-Willi Syndrome," Mayo Clinic, April 21, 2017, http://www.mayoclinic.org/diseases-conditions/prader-willi-syndrome/basics/symptoms/con-20028982.

3. Francis O. Walker, "Huntington's disease," *Lancet* 369, no. 9557 (January 20, 2007): 218–28, https://doi.org/10.1016/S0140-6736(07)60111-1, PMID 17240289.

4. Leslie A. Pray, "Transposons: the jumping genes," *Nature Education* 1, no. 1 (2008): 204.

5. J. C. Sanford, *Genetic Entropy & The Mystery of the Genome*, 3rd ed. (Waterloo, NY: FMS Publication), 42.

6. M. Jägerstad and K. Skog, "Genotoxicity of heat-processed foods," *Mutation Research* 574, no. 1–2 (July 2005): 156–72.

7. M. Q. Kemp et al., "Induction of the transferring receptor gene by benzo[a] pyrene in breast cancer MCF-7 cells: potential as a biomarker of PAH exposure," *Environmental & Molecular Mutagenesis* 47 (2006): 518–26.

8. B. Peterson et al., "Effects of prenatal exposure to air pollutants (polycyclic aromatic hydrocarbons) on the development of brain white matter, cognition, and behavior in later childhood," *Journal of the American Medical Association: Psychiatry* 72, no. 6 (2015): 531–40, https://doi.org/10.1001/jamapsychiatry.2015.57; F. P. Perera et al., "Prenatal polycyclic aromatic hydrocarbon (PAH) exposure and child behavior at age 6–7 years," *Environmental Health Perspectives* 120, no. 6 (2012): 921–26, https://doi.org/10.1289/ehp.1104315.

9. M. Valko, H. Morris, and M. T. Cronin, "Metals, toxicity and oxidative stress," *Current Medicinal Chemistry* 12, no. 10 (2005): 1161–1208, https://doi.org/10.2174/0929867053764635, PMID15892631.

10. N. Muñoz et al., "HPV in the etiology of human cancer," *Vaccine* 24, no. 3, supp. 3 (August 31, 2006): 1–10.

11. Sahaya Asirvatham, Rupali Yadav, and Hitesh Chaube, "Role of telomeres and telomerase in aging," *World Journal of Pharmaceutical Research* 4, no. 5 (2015): 697–708.

12. Lawrence S. Honig et al., "Association of shorter leukocyte telomere repeat length with dementia and mortality," *Archives of Neurology* 69, no. 10 (2012): 1332–39, https://doi.org/10.1001/archneurol.2012.1541.

13. K. Okudo et al., "Telomere length in the newborn," *Pediatric Research* 52 (2002): 377–81.

14. D. T. Eisenberg, M. G. Hayes, and C. W. Kuzawa, "Delayed paternal age of reproduction in humans is associated with longer telomeres across two generations of descendants," *Proceedings of the National Academy of Sciences of the*

United States of America 109 (2012): 10251–56; M. Kimura et al., "Offspring's leukocyte telomere length, paternal age, and telomere elongation in sperm," *PLOS Genetics* 4 (2008): e37.

15. A. Aviv, "Genetics of leukocyte telomere length and its role in atherosclerosis," *Mutation Research* 730 (2012): 68–74.

16. I. Shalev et al., "Exposure to violence during childhood is associated with telomere erosion from 5 to 10 years of age: a longitudinal study," *Molecular Psychiatry* 18 (2013): 576–81, https://doi.org/10.1038/mp.2012.32.

17. Elizabeth Fernandez, "Lifestyle Changes May Lengthen Telomeres, a Measure of Cell Aging," University of California, San Francisco, September 16, 2013, https://www.ucsf.edu/news/2013/09/108886/lifestyle-changes-may-lengthen-telomeres-measure-cell-aging.

18. Min Kyoung-Bok and Min Jin-Young, "Association between leukocyte telomere length and serum carotenoid in US adults," *European Journal of Nutrition* 56, no. 3 (April 2017): 1045–52.

19. D. Ornish et al., "Effect of comprehensive lifestyle changes on telomerase activity and telomere length in men with biopsy-proven low-risk prostate cancer: 5-year follow-up of a descriptive pilot study," *Lancet Oncology* 14, no. 11 (October 2013): 1112–20.

20. P. Sjögren et al., "Stand up for health—avoiding sedentary behaviour might lengthen your telomeres: secondary outcomes from a physical activity RCT in older people," *British Journal of Sports Medicine* 48 (September 3, 2014): 1407–9, https://doi.org/10.1136/bjsports-2013-093342, PMID 25185586.

21. T. Kanaya et al., "hTERT is a critical determinant of telomerase activity in renal-cell carcinoma," *International Journal of Cancer* 78, no. 5 (November 23, 1998): 539–43.

Chapter 5 Obesity and Aging

1. Deborah Summers, "No Excuses for Being Fat, Say Tories," *Guardian*, August 27, 2008, https://www.theguardian.com/politics/2008/aug/27/conservatives.health1.

2. Furukawa Shigetada et al., "Increased oxidative stress in obesity and its impact on metabolic syndrome," *Journal of Clinical Investigation* 114, no. 12 (2004): 1752–61.

3. A. E. Silver et al., "Overweight and obese humans demonstrate increased vascular endothelial NAD(P)H oxidase-p47(phox) expression and evidence of endothelial oxidative stress," *Circulation* 115, no. 5 (February 6, 2007): 627–37. See also A. S. Greenberg et al., "Obesity and the role of adipose tissue in inflammation and metabolism," *American Journal of Clinical Nutrition* 83, no. 2 (February 2006): 461S–65S; K. M. Pou et al., "Visceral and subcutaneous adipose tissue volumes are cross-sectionally related to markers of inflammation and oxidative stress: the Framingham Heart Study," *Circulation* 116, no. 11 (September 11, 2007): 1234–41.

4. H. Stein et al., "A commonly carried allele of the obesity-related FTO gene is associated with reduced brain volume in the healthy elderly," *Proceedings of*

the *National Academy of Sciences of the United States of America* 107, no. 18 (May 4, 2010): 8404–9.

5. American Heart Association Statistical Fact Sheet 2013, http://www.heart.org/idc/groups/heart-public/@wcm/@sop/@smd/documents/downloadable/ucm_319574.pdf.

6. G. Copinschi, "Metabolic and endocrine effects of sleep deprivation," *Essential Psychopharmacology* 6, no. 6 (2005): 341–47, PMID 16459757.

7. Institute of Medicine, *Sleep Disorders and Sleep Deprivation: An Unmet Public Health Problem* (Washington, DC: The National Academies Press, 2006), quoted from http://www.cdc.gov/features/dssleep/index.html#References.

8. "Insufficient Sleep Is a Public Health Problem," Centers for Disease Control and Prevention (2015), http://www.cdc.gov/features/dssleep/index.html#References.

9. J. Davis, "The Toll of Sleep Loss in America," WebMD, 2011, http://www.webmd.com/sleep-disorders/features/toll-of-sleep-loss-in-america.

10. A. Alvheim et al., "Dietary linoleic acid elevates endogenous 2-AG and anandamide and induces obesity," *Obesity* 20, no. 10 (2012): 1984–94.

11. P. Kidd, "Omega-3 DHA and EPA for cognition, behavior, and mood: clinical findings and structural functional synergies with cell membrane phospholipids," *Alternative Medicine Review* 12, no. 3 (2007).

12. S. Doughman et al., "Omega-3 fatty acids for nutrition and medicine: considering microalgae oil as a vegetarian source of EPA and DHA," *Current Diabetes Reviews* 3, no. 3 (August 2007): 198–203(6). See also J. T. Brenna et al., "α-Linolenic acid supplementation and conversion to n-3 long-chain polyunsaturated fatty acids in humans," *Prostaglandins, Leukotrienes & Essential Fatty Acids* 80, nos. 2–3 (February–March 2009): 85–91; L. M. Arterburn, "Human distribution of docosahexaenoic acid and eicosapentaenoic acid," *Medscape General Medicine* 7, no. 4 (2005): 18, Medscape, http://www.medscape.org/viewarticle/514322_4; S. Dyall, "Long-chain omega-3 fatty acids and the brain: a review of the independent and shared effects of EPA, DPA and DHA," *Frontiers in Aging Neuroscience* 7 (April 21, 2015): 52, https://doi.org/10.3389/fnagi.2015.00052.

13. L. Zhang et al., "Exogenous plant MIR168a specifically targets mammalian LDLRAP1: evidence of cross-kingdom regulation by microRNA," *Cell Research* 22 (2012): 107–26.

14. A. Foss, "Growing Fatter on a GM Diet," ScienceNordic, July 17, 2012, http://sciencenordic.com/growing-fatter-gm-diet.

15. R. Ley et al., "Microbial ecology: human gut microbes associated with obesity," *Nature* 444 (December 21, 2006): 1022–23, https://doi.org/10.1038/4441022a.

16. H. Tilg and A. Kaser, "Gut microbiome, obesity, and metabolic dysfunction," *Journal of Clinical Investigation* 121, no. 6 (2011): 2126–32, https://doi.org/10.1172/JCI58109.

17. F. Thomas et al., "Environmental and gut Bacteroidetes: the food connection," *Frontiers in Microbiology* 2 (2011): 93.

18. Thomas et al., "Environmental and gut Bacteroidetes."

19. L. David et al., "Diet rapidly and reproducibly alters the human gut microbiome," *Nature* 505 (January 23, 2014): 559–63; G. Wu et al., "Linking long-term

dietary patterns with gut microbial enterotypes," *Science* 334, no. 6052 (October 7, 2011): 105–8.

20. C. B. de La Serre et al., "Propensity to high-fat diet-induced obesity in rats is associated with changes in the gut microbiota and gut inflammation," *American Journal of Physiology: Gastrointestinal and Liver Physiology* 299, no. 2 (July 28, 2010): G440–48.

21. Herbert Tilg and Arthur Kaser, "Gut microbiome, obesity, and metabolic dysfunction," *Journal of Clinical Investigation* 121, no. 6 (June 2011): 2126–32, https://doi.org/10.1172/JCI58109.

22. K. Harris et al., "Is the gut microbiota a new factor contributing to obesity and its metabolic disorders?," *Journal of Obesity* 2012 (2012), https://doi.org/10.1155/2012/879151.

23. L. Lynch et al., "iNKT cells induce FGF21 for thermogenesis and are required for maximal weight loss in GLP1 therapy," *Cell Metabolism* 24, no. 3 (September 13, 2016): 510–19, http://dx.doi.org/10.1016/j.cmet.2016.08.003; J. Lukens et al., "Fat chance: not much against NKT cells," *Immunity* 37, no. 3 (September 21, 2012): 574–87.

24. L. C. Wieland Brown et al., "Production of α-Galactosylceramide by a prominent member of the human gut microbiota," *PLOS Biology* 11, no. 7 (2013): e1001610, https://doi.org/10.1371/journal.pbio.1001610.

25. B. T. Heijmans et al., "Persistent epigenetic differences associated with prenatal exposure to famine in humans," *Proceedings of the National Academy of Sciences of the United States of America* 105, no. 44 (November 4, 2008): 17046–49.

26. I. Parra-Rojas et al., "Adenovirus-36 seropositivity and its relation with obesity and metabolic profile in children," *International Journal of Endocrinology* 2013 (2013), http://dx.doi.org/10.1155/2013/463194.

27. M. Blüher et al., "Adipose tissue selective insulin receptor knockout protects against obesity and obesity-related glucose intolerance," *Developmental Cell* 3, no. 1 (July 2002): 25–38; M. Blüher et al., "Extended longevity in mice lacking the insulin receptor in adipose tissue," *Science* 299, no. 5606 (January 24, 2003): 572–74.

Chapter 6 Sugar, Oxidation, and Aging

1. S. L. Archer et al., "Relationship between changes in dietary sucrose and high density lipoprotein cholesterol: the CARDIA study. Coronary artery risk development in young adults," *Annals of Epidemiology* 8 (October 1998): 433–38.

2. Q. Yang et al., "Added sugar intake and cardiovascular diseases mortality among US adults," *Journal of the American Medical Association: Internal Medicine* 174, no. 4 (2014): 516–24; B. Howard et al., "Sugar and cardiovascular disease: a statement for healthcare professionals from the Committee on Nutrition of the Council on Nutrition, Physical Activity, and Metabolism of the American Heart Association," *Circulation* 106 (2002): 523–27.

3. R. Agrawal et al., "'Metabolic syndrome' in the brain: deficiency in omega-3 fatty acid exacerbates dysfunctions in insulin receptor signalling and cognition," *Journal of Physiology* 590, no. 10 (May 2012): 2485–99.

4. Alice G. Walton, "How Much Sugar Are Americans Eating," Forbes, August 30, 2012, http://www.forbes.com/sites/alicegwalton/2012/08/30/how-much-sugar -are-americans-eating-infographic/#5a72e9ef1f71.

5. C. Leung et al., "Soda and cell aging: associations between sugar-sweetened beverage consumption and leukocyte telomere length in healthy adults from the National Health and Nutrition Examination Surveys," *American Journal of Public Health* 104, no. 12 (December 2014): 2425–31, http://ajph.aphapublications.org /doi/abs/10.2105/AJPH.2014.302151.

6. J. E. Beilharz et al., "Short-term exposure to a diet high in fat and sugar, or liquid sugar, selectively impairs hippocampal-dependent memory, with differential impacts on inflammation," *Behavioural Brain Research* 306 (June 1, 2016): 1–7.

7. K. Rapinski, "Face Facts: Too Much Sugar Can Cause Wrinkles," NBC News report with dermatologist Dr. Frederick Brandt, http://www.nbcnews.com /id/21257751/ns/health-skin_and_beauty/t/face-facts-too-much-sugar-can-cause -wrinkles/#.V20eGZMrI0o; K. Mizutari et al., "Photo-enhanced modification of human skin elastin in actinic elastosis by N^ϵ-(carboxymethyl)lysine, one of the glycoxidation products of the Maillard reaction," *Journal of Investigative Dermatology* 108, no. 5 (May 1997): 797–802.

8. Alison Goldin et al., "Advanced glycation end products: sparking the development of diabetic vascular injury," *Circulation* 114 (August 2006): 597–605, http://circ.ahajournals.org/content/114/6/597.full.

9. R. Spangler et al., "Opiate-like effects of sugar on gene expression in reward areas of the rat brain," *Molecular Brain Research* 124, no. 2 (May 19, 2004): 134–42.

10. C. Blais et al., "Effect of dietary sodium restriction on taste responses to sodium chloride: a longitudinal study," *American Journal of Clinical Nutrition* 44, no. 2 (August 1986): 232–43.

11. X. Guo X et al., "Sweetened beverages, coffee, and tea and depression risk among older US adults," *PLOS ONE* 9, no. 4 (April 17, 2014): e94715, https:// doi.org/10.1371/journal.pone.0094715.

12. C. McGartland et al., "Carbonated soft drink consumption and bone mineral density in adolescence: the Northern Ireland Young Hearts project," *Journal of Bone and Mineral Research* 18, no. 9 (September 2003): 1563–69.

13. K. Tucker et al., "Colas, but not other carbonated beverages, are associated with low bone mineral density in older women: the Framingham Osteoporosis Study," *American Journal of Clinical Nutrition* 84, no. 4 (October 2006): 936–42.

14. M. Schultze et al., "Sugar-sweetened beverages, weight gain, and incidence of type 2 diabetes in young and middle-aged women," *Journal of the American Medical Association* 292, no. 8 (2004): 927–34, https://doi.org/10.1001/jama.292 .8.927.

15. S. Fowler et al., "Fueling the obesity epidemic? Artificially sweetened beverage use and long-term weight gain," *Obesity* 16, no. 8 (August 2008): 1894–1900.

16. A. Sánchez-Villegas et al., "Fast-food and commercial baked goods consumption and the risk of depression," *Public Health Nutrition* 15, no. 3 (2012): 424–32.

17. B. Martin et al., "Caloric restriction and intermittent fasting: two potential diets for successful brain aging," *Ageing Research Reviews* 5, no. 3 (August 2006):

332–53; G. Roth et al., "Biomarkers of caloric restriction may predict longevity in humans," *Science* 297, no. 5582 (August 2002): 811.

18. A. Csiszar et al., "Anti-oxidative and anti-inflammatory vasoprotective effects of caloric restriction in aging: role of circulating factors and SIRT1," *Mechanisms of Ageing and Development* 130, no. 8 (August 2009): 518–27.

19. Dale Bredesen, "Reversal of cognitive decline: a novel therapeutic program," *Aging* 6, no. 9 (September 2014): 707–17.

20. G. L. Bowman et al., "Nutrient biomarker patterns, cognitive function, and MRI measures of brain aging," *Neurology* 78, no. 4 (January 24, 2012): 241–49, https://doi.org/10.1212/WNL.0b013e3182436598.

21. J. Pottala et al., "Higher RBC EPA + DHA corresponds with larger total brain and hippocampal volumes," *Neurology* 82, no. 5 (February 4, 2014): 435–42.

22. Simon C. Dyall, "Long-chain omega-3 fatty acids and the brain: a review of the independent and shared effects of EPA, DPA and DHA," *Frontiers in Aging Neuroscience* 7, no. 52 (April 21, 2015), https://doi.org/10.3389/fnagi.2015.00052.

23. H. Ren et al., "Omega-3 polyunsaturated fatty acids promote amyloid-β clearance from the brain through mediating the function of the glymphatic system," *FASEB Journal* (October 7, 2016), https://doi.org/10.1096/fj.201600896.

24. Dyall, "Long-chain omega-3 fatty acids and the brain."

Chapter 7 Tobacco, Illegal Substances, Alcohol, and Aging

1. Rebecca Swanner et al., *Best You Ever* (New York: Simon and Shuster, 2011), https://books.google.com/books?id=XO_sDQAAQBAJ&pg=PT246&lpg =PT246&dq=The+Best+Way+to+Detoxify+is+to+Stop+Putting+Toxic +Things+into+the+Body&source=bl&ots=K3dLVJKhs_&sig=ZqHqbaLMLr PyCMCphMDxw7dHeVU&hl=en&sa=X&ved=0ahUKEwiny_HH773WAh WmE5oKHYsYCTwQ6AEIRDAG#v=onepage&q=The%20Best%20Way%20 to%20Detoxify%20is%20to%20Stop%20Putting%20Toxic%20Things%20into %20the%20Body&f=false.

2. D. Doshi et al., "Smoking and skin aging in identical twins," *Archives of Dermatology* 143, no. 12 (2007): 1543–46, https://doi.org/10.1001/archderm.143 .12.1543. Pictures of these twins can be seen at http://archderm.jamanetwork.com /article.aspx?articleid=654484.

3. S. Ramirez et al., "Methamphetamine disrupts blood-brain barrier function by induction of oxidative stress in brain endothelial cells," *Journal of Cerebral Blood Flow & Metabolism* 29, no. 12 (2009): 1933–45.

4. W. Sheng-Fan et al., "Involvement of oxidative stress-activated JNK signaling in the methamphetamine-induced cell death of human SH-SY5Y cells," *Toxicology* 246, nos. 2–3 (April 18, 2008): 234–41.

5. R. Little et al., "Fetal growth and moderate drinking in early pregnancy," *American Journal of Epidemiology* 123, no. 2 (1986): 270–78; P. Sampson et al., "Prenatal alcohol exposure, birthweight, and measures of child size from birth to 14 years," *American Journal of Public Health* 84, no. 9 (September 1994): 1421–28.

6. S. Sabia et al., "Alcohol consumption and cognitive decline in early old age," *Neurology* 82, no. 4 (January 28, 2014): 332–39; E. Handing et al., "Midlife alcohol consumption and risk of dementia over 43 years of follow-up: a population-based

study from the Swedish Twin Registry," *Journals of Gerontology: Series A* 70, no. 10 (October 1, 2015): 1248–54, https://doi.org/10.1093/gerona/glv038.

7. M. De Bellis et al., "Prefrontal cortex, thalamus, and cerebellar volumes in adolescents and young adults with adolescent-onset alcohol use disorders and comorbid mental disorders," *Alcoholism: Clinical and Experimental Research* 29, no. 9 (September 2005): 1590–1600.

8. B. Davis et al., "The alcohol paradox: light-to-moderate alcohol consumption, cognitive function, and brain volume," *Journals of Gerontology: Series A* 69, no. 12 (December 2014): 1528–35, https://doi.org/10.1093/gerona/glu092.

9. J. Patra et al., "Alcohol consumption and the risk of morbidity and mortality for different stroke types—a systematic review and meta-analysis," *Biomed Central Public Health* 10, no. 258 (May 18, 2010); S. Larsson et al., "Differing association of alcohol consumption with different stroke types: a systematic review and meta-analysis," *Biomed Central Medicine* 14, no. 178 (2016).

10. Handing et al., "Midlife alcohol consumption," https://doi.org/10.1093/gerona/glv038.

11. A. Waterhouse, "Wine phenolics," *Annals of the New York Academy of Sciences* 957 (May 2002): 21–36.

12. G. M. Halpern, "A celebration of wine: wine is medicine," *Inflammopharmacology* 16, no. 5 (October 2008): 240–44, https://doi.org/10.1007/s10787-008-8024-9. See also A. Dávalos et al., "Effects of red grape juice polyphenols in NADPH oxidase subunit expression in human neutrophils and mononuclear blood cells," *British Journal of Nutrition* 102, no. 8 (October 28, 2009): 1125–35, https://doi.org/10.1017/S0007114509382148; M. Sarr et al., "Red wine polyphenols prevent angiotensin II-induced hypertension and endothelial dysfunction in rats: role of NADPH oxidase," *Cardiovascular Research* 71, no. 4 (September 1, 2006): 794–802; M. Dohadwala et al., "Grapes and cardiovascular disease," *Journal of Nutrition* 139, no. 9 (September 2009): 1788S–93S; R. F. Guerrero et al., "Wine, resveratrol and health: a review," *National Product Communication* 4, no. 5 (May 2009): 635–58.

13. E. Lobe et al., "Is there an association between low-to-moderate alcohol consumption and risk of cognitive decline?," *American Journal of Epidemiology* 172, no. 6 (2010): 708–16, https://doi.org/10.1093/aje/kwq187.

14. The immediate effect of alcohol upon the brain is to interact with neuronal membranes, altering their function and causing a change in ionic balance (primarily, chloride ions that are negatively charged flow into the cells making the neurons more negatively charged and less likely to fire, thus sedating them), which results in the various symptoms of intoxication. However, alcohol also causes epigenetic changes in the brain that alter gene expression in the fear circuit (amygdala), which increase anxiety once the intoxication clears. Specifically, alcohol intoxication causes the production of a peptide, called Neuropeptide Y (NPY), in the amygdala that is also associated with the relaxing effect of intoxication. However, once the alcohol clears (intoxication is over) there is a rebound suppression of NPY, which causes the amygdala to be more active, increasing anxiety and cravings for alcohol. See B. Hwang et al., "Innate differences of neuropeptide Y (NPY) in hypothalamic nuclei and central nucleus of the amygdala between selectively bred rats with high and low alcohol preference," *Alcoholism:*

Clinical and Experimental Research 23, no. 6 (June 1999): 1023–30; C. Eva et al., "Modulation of neuropeptide Y and Y_1 receptor expression in the amygdala by fluctuations in the brain content of neuroactive steroids during ethanol drinking discontinuation in $Y_1R/LacZ$ transgenic mice," *Journal of Neurochemistry* 104 (2008): 1043–54; J. D. Olling et al., "Complex plastic changes in the neuropeptide Y system during ethanol intoxication and withdrawal in the rat brain," *Journal of Neuroscience Research* 87, no. 10 (August 1, 2009): 2386–97.

15. L. Zhu et al., "Characterization of gut microbiomes in nonalcoholic steatohepatitis (NASH) patients: a connection between endogenous alcohol and NASH," *Hepatology* 57, no. 2 (February 2013): 601–9. See also S. Nair et al., "Obesity and female gender increase breath ethanol concentration: potential implications for the pathogenesis of nonalcoholic steatohepatitis," *American Journal of Gastroenterology* 96 (2001): 1200–4; K. Cope et al., "Increased gastrointestinal ethanol production in obese mice: implications for fatty liver disease pathogenesis," *Gastroenterology* 119, no. 5 (November 2000): 1340–47.

Chapter 8 Exercise and Your Brain

1. Devin Tomb, "Self-Made Women Who Inspire: 4 Entrepreneurs Who Motivate," *Self*, January 5, 2015, https://www.self.com/story/selfmade-women-entrepreneurs-who-motivate.

2. *Poor Richard's Almanack* (1742), http://www.vlib.us/amdocs/texts/prichard42.html.

3. Extract from Thomas Jefferson to Martha Jefferson Randolph, Aix en Provence, March 28, 1787, Thomas Jefferson Foundation, http://tjrs.monticello.org/letter/1679.

4. Thomas Jefferson to Peter Carr, August 19, 1785, Thomas Jefferson Foundation, https://www.monticello.org/site/research-and-collections/exercise.

5. Jefferson to Carr, https://www.monticello.org/site/research-and-collections/exercise.

6. U. Kujala, "Evidence on the effects of exercise therapy in the treatment of chronic disease," *British Journal of Sports Medicine* 43 (2009): 550–55.

7. W. H. Ettinger Jr. et al., "A randomized trial comparing aerobic exercise and resistance exercise with a health education program in older adults with knee osteoarthritis. The Fitness Arthritis and Seniors Trial (FAST)," *Journal of the American Medical Association* 277, no. 1 (January 1, 1997): 25–31.

8. I. Helmark et al., "Exercise increases interleukin-10 levels both intra-articularly and peri-synovially in patients with knee osteoarthritis: a randomized controlled trial," *Arthritis Research & Therapy* 12, no. 4 (2010): R126, https://doi.org/10.1186/ar3064; F. Ribeiro et al., "Exercise training increases interleukin-10 after an acute myocardial infarction: a randomised clinical trial," *International Journal of Sports Medicine* 33, no. 3 (March 2012): 192–98, https://doi.org/10.1055/s-0031-1297959.

9. K. Jin et al., "Vascular endothelial growth factor (VEGF) stimulates neurogenesis in vitro and in vivo," *Proceedings of the National Academy of Sciences of the United States of America* 99, no. 18 (September 3, 2002): 11946–50; R. Molteni et al., "Voluntary exercise increases axonal regeneration from sensory

neurons," *Proceedings of the National Academy of Sciences of the United States of America* 101, no. 22 (June 1, 2004): 8473–78; M. Fahnestock et al., "The precursor pro-nerve growth factor is the predominant form of nerve growth factor in brain and is increased in Alzheimer's disease," *Molecular and Cellular Neuroscience* 18, no. 2 (August 2001): 210–20.

10. K. Erikson et al., "Exercise training increases size of hippocampus and improves memory," *Proceedings of the National Academy of Sciences of the United States of America* 108, no. 7 (February 2011): 3017–22.

11. K. Y. Liang et al., "Exercise and Alzheimer's disease biomarkers in cognitively normal older adults," *Annals of Neurology* 68 (2010): 311–18.

12. Liang et al., "Exercise and Alzheimer's disease biomarkers."

13. Liang et al., "Exercise and Alzheimer's disease biomarkers."

14. F. Middleton and P. Strick, "Basal ganglia output and cognition: evidence from anatomical, behavioral, and clinical studies," *Brain and Cognition* 42, no. 2 (March 2000): 183–200.

15. J. Schmahmann, "Disorders of the cerebellum: ataxia, dysmetria of thought, and the cerebellar cognitive affective syndrome," *Journal of Neuropsychiatry and the Clinical Neurosciences* 16, no. 3 (August 2004): 367–78.

16. C. Gaser et al., "Brain structures differ between musicians and non-musicians," *Journal of Neuroscience* 23, no. 27 (October 8, 2003): 9240–45.

17. S. Belleville et al., "Training-related brain plasticity in subjects at risk of developing Alzheimer's disease," *Brain* 134 (2011): 1623–34; S. M. Landau et al., "Association of lifetime cognitive engagement and low ß-amyloid deposition," *Archives of Neurology* 69 (2012): 623–29.

18. C. Bouchard et al., "Adverse metabolic response to regular exercise: Is it a rare or common occurrence?," *PLOS ONE* 7, no. 5 (2012): e37887, https://doi.org/10.1371/journal.pone.0037887.

19. A. Mastaloudis et al., "Oxidative stress in athletes during extreme endurance exercise," *Free Radical Biology and Medicine* 31, no. 7 (October 1, 2001): 911–22. See also S. Möhlenkamp et al., "Coronary atherosclerosis burden, but not transient troponin elevation, predicts long-term outcome in recreational marathon runners," *Basic Research in Cardiology* 109 (January 2014): 391, https://doi.org/10.1007/s00395-013-0391-8; J. O'Keefe et al., "Exercising for health and longevity vs peak performance: different regimens for different goals," *Mayo Clinic Proceedings* 89, no. 9 (September 2014): 1171–75.

20. T. Manini et al., "Physical activity and maintaining physical function in older adults," *British Journal of Sports Medicine* 43 (2009): 28–31.

Chapter 9 Sleep and Your Brain

1. "Insufficient Sleep Is a Public Health Problem," Centers for Disease Control and Prevention, 2015, http://www.cdc.gov/Features/dsSleep/index.html.

2. H. Colten and B. Altevogt, *Sleep Disorders and Sleep Deprivation: An Unmet Public Health Problem* (Washington, DC: The National Academies Press, 2006).

3. "Unhealthy Sleep-Related Behaviors," *Centers for Disease Control and Prevention Morbidity and Mortality Weekly Report* 60, no. 8 (March 4, 2011), http://www.cdc.gov/mmwr/PDF/wk/mm6008.pdf.

4. "Drowsy Driving and Automobile Crashes," National Highway Traffic Safety Administration, accessed February 10, 2011, http://www.nhtsa.gov/people /injury/drowsy_driving1/Drowsy.html#NCSDR/NHTSA.

5. L. Xie et al., "Sleep drives metabolite clearance from the adult brain," *Science* 342, no. 6156 (October 18, 2013): 373–77, https://doi.org/10.1126/science.1241224.

6. "Excessive Sleepiness: How Much Sleep Do Babies and Kids Need?," National Sleep Foundation, https://sleepfoundation.org/excessivesleepiness/content /how-much-sleep-do-babies-and-kids-need.

7. C. A. Schoenborn and P. F. Adams, "Health behaviors of adults: United States, 2005–2007," National Center for Health Statistics, *Vital Health Statistic Series* 10, no. 245 (2010).

8. "Youth Risk Behavior Surveillance—United States, 2009," *Centers for Disease Control and Prevention Morbidity and Mortality Weekly Report* 59 (June 4, 2010), SS-5.

9. "School Start Time and Sleep," National Sleep Foundation, http://www .sleepfoundation.org/article/sleep-topics/school-start-time-and-sleep.

10. N. Dumay, "Sleep not just protects memories against forgetting, it also makes them more accessible," *Cortex* 74 (January 2016): 289–96.

11. F. Gu et al., "Total and cause-specific mortality of U.S. nurses working rotating night shifts," *American Journal of Preventive Medicine* 48, no. 3 (March 2015): 241–52.

12. John Peever, Pierre-Hervé Luppi, and Jacques Montplaisir, "Breakdown in REM sleep circuitry underlies REM sleep behavior disorder," *Trends in Neurosciences* 37, no. 5 (May 2014): 279–88.

13. D. L. Bliwise, "Sleep disorders in Alzheimer's disease and other dementias," *Clinical Cornerstone* 6, supp. 1A (2004): S16–28.

14. M. Nishida et al., "REM sleep, prefrontal theta, and the consolidation of human emotional memory," *Cerebral Cortex* 19, no. 5 (May 2009): 1158–66.

15. W. Brown, "Broken sleep may be natural sleep," *Psychiatric Times* (March 1, 2007), http://www.psychiatrictimes.com/display/article/10168/55271.

16. A. Pariente et al., "The benzodiazepine-dementia disorders link: current state of knowledge," *CNS Drugs* 30, no. 1 (January 2016): 1–7, https://doi.org /10.1007/s40263-015-0305-4.

17. G. Chapouthier and P. Venault, "GABA-A receptor complex and memory processes," *Current Topics in Medicinal Chemistry* 2, no. 8 (August 1, 2002): 841–51; I. Izquierdo et al., "Post-training down-regulation of memory consolidation by a GABA-A mechanism in the amygdala modulated by endogenous benzodiazepines," *Behavioral and Neural Biology* 54, no. 2 (September 1990): 105–9.

18. D. Wheatley, "Effects of Drugs on Sleep," *Psychopharmacology of Sleep*, ed. D. Wheatley (New York: Raven Press, 1981), 153–76.

19. M. Ratini, "7 Ways Sleep Apnea Can Hurt Your Health," WebMD, May, 2, 2016, http://www.webmd.com/sleep-disorders/sleep-apnea/sleep-apnea-con ditions#1.

20. N. Canessa et al., "Obstructive sleep apnea: Brain structural changes and neurocognitive function before and after treatment," *American Journal of Respiratory and Critical Care Medicine* 183, no. 10 (May 15, 2011): 1419–26, https:// doi.org/10.1164/rccm.201005-0693OC.

21. "Caffeine for the Sustainment of Mental Task Performance: Formulations for Military Operations," National Academies of Sciences, Engineering, and Medicine (Washington, DC: National Academies Press, 2001), https://doi.org/10.17226/10219.

22. S. Brand et al., "High self-perceived exercise exertion before bedtime is associated with greater objectively assessed sleep efficiency," *Sleep Medicine* 15, no. 9 (September 2014): 1031–36.

Chapter 10 A Vacation in Time

1. M. Kivimäki et al., "Long working hours and risk of coronary heart disease and stroke: a systematic review and meta-analysis of published and unpublished data for 603,838 individuals," *Lancet* 386, no. 10005 (October 31–November 6, 2015): 1739–46.

2. T. Hoshuyama, "Overwork and its health effects—current status and future approach regarding Karoshi," *Sangyo Eisegaku Zasshi (Journal of Occupational Health)* 45, no. 5 (2003): 187–93.

3. M. Irie et al., "Relationships between perceived workload, stress and oxidative DNA damage," *International Archives of Occupational and Environmental Health* 74, no. 2 (2001): 153–57, https://doi.org/10.1007/s004200000209.

4. E. Epel et al., "Meditation and vacation effects have an impact on disease-associated molecular phenotypes," *Translational Psychiatry* 6 (2016): e880, https://doi.org/10.1038/tp.2016.164.

5. D. Buettner, "Lessons for Living Longer from the People Who've Lived the Longest," Blue Zones, 2008, http://www.bluezones.com/live-longer/education/expeditions/loma-linda-california/.

6. E. Morita et al., "Psychological effects of forest environments on healthy adults: shinrin-yoku (forest-air bathing, walking) as a possible method of stress reduction," *Public Health* 121, no. 1 (January 2007): 54–63.

7. J. Lee et al., "Effect of forest bathing on physiological and psychological responses in young Japanese male subjects," *Public Health* 125, no. 2 (February 2011): 93–100.

8. U. Stigsdotter et al., "Health promoting outdoor environments—associations between green space, and health, health-related quality of life and stress based on a Danish national representative survey," *Scandinavian Journal of Public Health* 38, no. 4 (June 2010): 411–17.

9. L. O'Brien, "Learning outdoors: the Forest School approach," *Education 3–13* 37, no. 1 (2009): 45–60; L. O'Brien, "Forest School and its impact on young children: case studies in Britain," *Urban Forestry and Urban Greening* 6, no. 4 (November 2007): 249–65.

10. H. I. Kruppa, "Health effects caused by noise: evidence in the literature from the past 25 years," *Noise Health* 6 (2004): 5–13.

11. W. Babisch, "Road traffic noise and cardiovascular risk," *Noise Health* 10, no. 38 (January–March 2008): 27–33.

12. V. Regecová, "Effects of urban noise pollution on blood pressure and heart rate in preschool children," *Journal of Hypertension* 13, no. 4 (April 1995): 405–12.

13. M. Haines et al., "Chronic aircraft noise exposure, stress responses, mental health and cognitive performance in school children," *Psychological Medicine* 31, no. 2 (2001): 265–77, https://doi.org/10.1017/S0033291701003282.

14. John P. O'Reardon et al., "Efficacy and safety of transcranial magnetic stimulation in the acute treatment of major depression: a multisite randomized controlled trial," *Biological Psychiatry* 62 (2007): 1208–16.

15. P. Sokal and K. Sokal, "The neuromodulative role of earthing," *Medical Hypotheses* 77, no. 5 (November 2011): 824–26.

16. J. L. Oschman, "Perspective: assume a spherical cow: the role of free or mobile electrons in bodywork, energetic and movement therapies," *Journal of Bodywork and Movement Therapies* 12, no. 1 (2008): 40–57.

17. J. L. Oschman, "Charge transfer in the living matrix," *Journal of Bodywork and Movement Therapies* 13, no. 3 (2009): 215–28.

18. J. L. Oschman et al., "The effects of grounding (earthing) on inflammation, the immune response, wound healing, and prevention and treatment of chronic inflammatory and autoimmune diseases," *Journal of Inflammation Research* 8 (2015): 83–96.

19. G. Chevalier et al., "One-hour contact with the Earth's surface (grounding) improves inflammation and blood flow—a randomized, double-blind, pilot study," *Health* 7, no. 8 (August 2015): 1022–59.

20. G. Chevalier et al., "Earthing: health implications of reconnecting the human body to the Earth's surface electrons," *Journal of Environmental and Public Health* 2012 (2012), https://doi.org/10.1155/2012/291541.

21. H. Cohen-Cline, E. Turkheimer, and G. Duncan, "Access to green space, physical activity and mental health: a twin study," *Journal of Epidemiology and Community Health* 69, no. 6 (2015): 523–29, https://doi.org/10.1136/jech-2014 -204667.

22. J. Barton and J. Pretty, "What is the best dose of nature and green exercise for improving mental health? A multi-study analysis," *Environmental Science & Technology* 44, no.10 (2010): 3947–55.

23. Q. Li et al., "Acute effects of walking in forest environments on cardiovascular and metabolic parameters," *European Journal of Applied Physiology* 111, no. 11 (November 2011): 2845–53, https://doi.org/10.1007/s00421-011-1918-z; V. Gladwell et al., "The great outdoors: how a green exercise environment can benefit all," *Extreme Physiology & Medicine* 2, no. 3 (2013), https://doi.org/10 .1186/2046-7648-2-3.

24. V. Gladwell et al., "The effects of views of nature on autonomic control," *European Journal of Applied Physiology* 112, no. 9 (September 2012): 3379–86.

25. H. Hasan and T. Hasan, "Laugh yourself into a healthier person: a cross cultural analysis of the effects of varying levels of laughter on health," *International Journal of Medical Sciences* 6, no. 4 (2009): 200–211.

26. Hasan and Hasan, "Laugh yourself into a healthier person," referencing vascular medicine. See also "Watching funny movies boosts blood flow to the heart," Health & Medicine Week, 1660 (2006), Research Library database, document ID 980266611.

27. S. A. Tan et al., "Humor, as an adjunct therapy in cardiac rehabilitation, attenuates catecholamines and myocardial infarction recurrence," *Advances in Mind-Body Medicine* 22, nos. 3–4 (2007): 8–12.

28. L. S. Berk, S. A. Tan, and W. F. Fry, "Eustress of humor associated laughter modulates specific immune system components," *Annals of Behavioral Medicine* 15, no. 11 (1993); L. S. Berk et al., "Eustress of mirthful laughter modifies natural killer cell activity," *Clinical Research* 37, no. 1 (1989): 115A.

Chapter 11 Our Beliefs and Aging

1. E. Mark, "Religion in Ancient China," Ancient History Encyclopedia, April 21, 2016, http://www.ancient.eu/article/891/.

2. J. Grehan, "Smoking and 'early modern' sociability: the great tobacco debate in the Ottoman Middle East (seventeenth to eighteenth centuries)," *American Historical Review* 111, no. 5 (December 2006): 1352–77. See also S. A. Dickson, *Panacea or Precious Bane. Tobacco in 16th Century Literature* (New York: New York Public Library, 1954); J. E. Brookes, *The Mighty Leaf: Tobacco Through the Centuries* (Boston: Little, Brown, 1952); G. G. Stewart, "A history of the medicinal use of tobacco 1492–1860," *Medical History* 11 (1967): 228–68; A. Charlton, "Medicinal uses of tobacco in history," *Journal of the Royal Society of Medicine* 97, no. 6 (June 2004): 292–96.

3. Gilbert R. Seigworth, MD, "Bloodletting over the centuries," *New York State Journal of Medicine* (December 1980), http://www.pbs.org/video/bloodletting-blisters-and-the-mystery-of-washington-s-death-1425939074/.

4. J. Haller, "American Medicine in Transition 1840–1910," *Indiana Magazine of History* 77, no. 4 (1981): 387–89.

5. H. Benson et al., "The placebo effect: a neglected asset in the care of patients," *Journal of the American Medical Association* 232, no. 12 (1975): 1225–27.

6. "This Day in History: October 30, 1938: Welles Scares Nation," History, http://www.history.com/this-day-in-history/welles-scares-nation.

7. Antonio Favaro, ed. (1890–1909), *Le Opere di Galileo Galilei, Edizione Nazionale* [*The Works of Galileo Galilei, National Edition*] (Florence: Barbera, 1900), 10:423.

8. "Doctor to Legislators: Refusing Medical Care Isn't Religious Freedom," *NBC News*, March 9, 2015, http://www.nbcnews.com/health/kids-health/doctor-legislators-refusing-medical-care-isnt-religious-freedom-n320031.

9. Jason Wilson, "Letting Them Die: Parents Refuse Medical Help for Children in the Name of Christ," *Guardian*, April 13, 2016, https://www.theguardian.com/us-news/2016/apr/13/followers-of-christ-idaho-religious-sect-child-mortality-refusing-medical-help.

10. A. H. Miller et al., "Inflammation and its discontents: the role of cytokines in the pathophysiology of major depression," *Biological Psychiatry* 65, no. 9 (2009): 732–41. See also S. A. Everson et al., "Depressive symptoms and increased risk of stroke mortality over a 29-year period," *Archives of Internal Medicine* 158 (1998): 1133–38; W. W. Eaton et al., "The influence of educational attainment on depression and risk of type 2 diabetes," *Diabetes Care* 19, no. 10 (1996): 1097–102; A. E. Yazici et al., "Bone mineral density in premenopausal women with major

depression," *Joint Bone Spine* 72 (2005): 540–43; J. S. Saczynski, "Depressive symptoms and the risk of dementia," *Neurology* 75, no. 1 (July 6, 2010): 35–41.

11. J. H. Hay, "A British Medical Association lecture on the significance of a raised blood pressure," *British Medical Journal* 2, no. 3679 (July 11, 1931): 43–47, https://doi.org/10.1136/bmj.2.3679.43, PMC 2314188, PMID 20776269.

12. Paul Dudley White, *Heart Disease*, 2nd ed. (New York: MacMillan Co., 1937), 326.

13. Wikipedia, s.v. "Spontaneous generation," last modified October 23, 2017, 15:34, https://en.wikipedia.org/wiki/Spontaneous_generation.

14. Wikipedia, s.v. "Abiogenesis," last modified November 28, 2017, 20:44, https://en.wikipedia.org/wiki/Abiogenesis.

15. Richard Dawkins, *The God Delusion* (Boston: Houghton Mifflin, 2006), 51.

16. If the reader is interested in a greater discussion of and the historical evidence for this assertion, I would refer them to my book *The God-Shaped Heart: How Correctly Understanding God's Love Transforms Us* (Grand Rapids: Baker Books, 2017).

17. Nancy Pearcey, *Finding Truth: 5 Principles for Unmasking Atheism, Secularism, and Other God Substitutes* (Ontario, Canada: David C. Cook Publishing, 2015), 25.

18. Pearcey, *Finding Truth*, 26.

19. Lee-Fay Low, Fleur Harrison, and Steven M. Lackersteen, "Does personality affect risk for dementia? A systematic review and meta-analysis," *American Journal of Geriatric Psychiatry* 21, no. 8 (August 2013): 713–28.

20. E. Langer, *Counterclockwise: Mindful Health and the Power of Possibility* (New York: Ballantine, 2009).

21. E. Kim et al., "Optimism and cause-specific mortality: a prospective cohort study," *American Journal of Epidemiology* 185, no. 1 (January 2017): 21–29, https://doi.org/10.1093/aje/kww182.

Chapter 12 Mental Stress and Aging

1. Y. K. Kim et al., "Cytokine imbalance in the pathophysiology of major depressive disorder," *Progress in Neuro-Psychopharmacology & Biological Psychiatry* 31, no. 5 (June 30, 2007): 1044–53. See also D. Musselman et al., "The relationship of depression to cardiovascular disease," *Archives of General Psychiatry* 55, no. 7 (1998): 580–92; A. H. Miller et al., "Inflammation and its discontents: the role of cytokines in the pathophysiology of major depression," *Biological Psychiatry* 65, no. 9 (2009): 732–41; S. Alesci et al., "Major depression is associated with significant diurnal elevations in plasma interleukin-6 levels, a shift of its circadian rhythm, and loss of physiological complexity in its secretion: clinical implications," *Journal of Clinical Endocrinology & Metabolism* 90, no. 5 (2005): 2522–30.

2. A. O'Donovan et al., "Pessimism correlates with leukocyte telomere shortness and elevated interleukin-6 in post-menopausal women," *Brain, Behavior, and Immunity* 23, no. 4 (May 2009): 446–49, https://doi.org/10.1016/j.bbi.2008.11.006.

3. B. R. Levy et al., "Longevity increased by positive self-perceptions of aging," *Journal of Personality and Social Psychology* 83 (2002): 261–70.

4. A. Danese et al., "Adverse childhood experiences and adult risk factors for age-related disease: depression, inflammation, and clustering of metabolic risk markers," *Archives of Pediatric & Adolescent Medicine* 163, no. 12 (2009): 1135–43. See also J. Bick et al., "Childhood adversity and DNA methylation of genes involved in the hypothalamus-pituitary-adrenal axis and immune system: whole-genome and candidate-gene associations," *Development & Psychopathology* 24, no. 4 (November 2012): 1417–25; J. Carroll et al., "Childhood abuse, parental warmth, and adult multisystem biological risk in the Coronary Artery Risk Development in Young Adults study," *Proceedings of the National Academy of Sciences of the United States of America* 110, no. 42 (October 15, 2013): 17149–53; M. Kelly-Irving et al., "Adverse childhood experiences and premature all-cause mortality," *European Journal of Epidemiology* 28, no. 9 (2013): 721–34; L. Gilbert et al., "Childhood adversity and adult chronic disease," *American Journal of Preventive Medicine* 48, no. 3 (March 2015): 345–49.

5. R. Lund, "Stressful social relations and mortality: a prospective cohort study," *Journal of Epidemiology & Community Health* 68, no. 8, https://doi.org/10.1136/jech-2013-203675.

6. S. W. Cole et al., "Social regulation of gene expression in human leukocytes," *Genome Biology* 8, no. 9 (2007): R189.

7. S. W. Cole et al., "Transcript origin analysis identifies antigen-presenting cells as primary targets of socially regulated gene expression in leukocytes," *Proceedings of the National Academy of Sciences of the United States of America* 108, no. 7: 3080–85.

8. N. J. Donovan et al., "Association of higher cortical amyloid burden with loneliness in cognitively normal older adults," *Journal of the American Medical Association: Psychiatry* 73, no. 12 (December 2016): 1230–37, https://doi.org/10.1001/jamapsychiatry.2016.2657.

9. M. B. Ospina et al., "Meditation practices for health: state of the research," *Evidence Report/Technology Assessment* 155 (June 2007): 1–263. See also P. Grossman et al., "Mindfulness-based stress reduction and health benefits: a meta-analysis," *Journal of Psychosomatic Research* 57, no. 1 (2004): 35–43; S. G. Hofmann et al., "The effect of mindfulness-based therapy on anxiety and depression: a meta-analytic review," *Journal of Consulting & Clinical Psychology* 78 (2010): 169–83; E. Bohlmeijer, R. Prenger, and E. Taal, "The effects of mindfulness-based stress reduction therapy on mental health of adults with a chronic medical disease: a meta-analysis," *Journal of Psychosomatic Research* 68, no. 6 (2010): 539–44; T. Kamei et al., "Decrease in serum cortisol during yoga exercise is correlated with α wave activation," *Perceptual & Motor Skills* 90, no. 3, pt. 1 (2000): 1027–32.

10. A. Newberg and Mark R. Waldman, *How God Changes Your Brain: Breakthrough Findings from a Leading Neuroscientist* (New York: Random House, 2009), 27–32, 53.

11. S. Post, *Altruism and Health Perspectives from Empirical Research* (New York: Oxford University Press, 2007), 22, 26.

Chapter 13 Love and Death

1. I. Yalom, *Existential Psychotherapy* (New York: Basic Books, 1980), 29.

2. Yalom, *Existential Psychotherapy*, 41.

3. Anders Andrén,"Behind 'heathendom': archaeological studies of Old Norse religion," *Scottish Archaeological Journal* 27, no. 2 (January 1, 2005): 105–38.

4. Richard Cavendish and Trevor Oswald Ling, *Mythology: An Illustrated Encyclopedia* (New York: Rizzoli, 1980), 40–45.

5. Jayaram V., "Death and Afterlife in Hinduism," Hinduwebsite.com, http://www.hinduwebsite.com/hinduism/h_death.asp.

6. "Islamic Beliefs about the Afterlife," ReligionFacts, March 17, 2015, accessed December 19, 2016, www.religionfacts.com/islam/afterlife.

7. Timothy Jennings, *The Remedy: A New Testament Expanded Paraphrase in Everyday English* (Chattanooga: Lennox Publishing, 2015).

Chapter 14 Pathological Aging

1. M. Prince et al., "The global prevalence of dementia: a systematic review and metaanalysis," *Alzheimers Dementia* 9, no. 1 (January 2013): 63–75.e2, https://doi.org/10.1016/j.jalz.2012.11.007.

2. Alzheimer's Association, "2014 Alzheimer's Disease Fact and Figures," *Alzheimer's & Dementia* 10, no. 2, http://www.alz.org/downloads/facts_figures_2014.pdf.

3. H. Ren et al., "Omega-3 polyunsaturated fatty acids promote amyloid-β clearance from the brain through mediating the function of the glymphatic system," *FASEB Journal* 31, no. 1 (January 2017): 282–93, https://doi.org/10.1096/fj.201600896.

4. L. D. Plant et al., "The production of amyloid beta peptide is a critical requirement for the viability of central neurons," *Journal of Neuroscience* 23, no. 13 (2003): 5531–35.

5. Chuang-Chung Lee et al., "A three-stage kinetic model of amyloid fibrillation," *Biophysical Journal* 92, no. 10 (May 15, 2007): 3448–58.

6. B. Su et al., "Oxidative stress signaling in Alzheimer's disease," *Current Alzheimer Research* 5, no. 6 (December 2008): 525–32.

7. H. G. Lee et al., "Challenging the amyloid cascade hypothesis: senile plaques and amyloid-beta as protective adaptations to Alzheimer disease," *Annals of the New York Academy of Sciences* 1019 (2004): 1–4; M. A. Smith et al., "Metabolic, metallic, and mitotic sources of oxidative stress in Alzheimer disease," *Antioxidants & Redox Signaling* 2 (2000): 413–20; C. A. Rottkamp et al., "The state versus amyloid-beta: the trial of the most wanted criminal in Alzheimer disease," *Peptides* 23 (2002): 1333–41.

8. T. Bird, "Early-onset familial Alzheimer disease," *GeneReviews*, last modified October 18, 2012, https://www.ncbi.nlm.nih.gov/books/NBK1236/.

9. "Alzheimer's Disease Fact Sheet," National Institute on Aging, https://www.nia.nih.gov/alzheimers/publication/alzheimers-disease-genetics-fact-sheet.

10. N. Ghebranious et al., "Detection of *ApoE E2, E3* and *E4* alleles using MALDI-TOF mass spectrometry and the homogeneous mass-extend technology," *Nucleic Acids Research* 33, no. 17 (January 2005): e149, https://doi.org/10.1093/nar/gni155, PMC 1243648, PMID 16204452. See also L. Zuo et al., "Variation at *APOE* and *STH* loci and Alzheimer's disease," *Behavioral & Brain Functions* 2, no. 13

(April 7, 2006), https://doi.org/10.1186/1744-9081-2-13, PMC 1526745, PMID 16603077; J. L. Breslow et al., "Studies of familial type III hyperlipoproteinemia using as a genetic marker the apoE phenotype E2/2," *Journal of Lipid Research* 23, no. 8 (1982): 1224–35, PMID 7175379; F. Civeira et al., "Apo E variants in patients with type III hyperlipoproteinemia," *Atherosclerosis* 127, no. 2 (1996): 273–82, https://doi.org/10.1016/S0021-9150(96)05969-2, PMID 9125318; R. W. Mahley, "Apolipoprotein E: cholesterol transport protein with expanding role in cell biology," *Science* 240, no. 4852 (April 1988): 622–30, https://doi.org/10.1126/science.3283935, PMID 3283935; E. H. Corder et al., "Gene dose of apolipoprotein E type 4 allele and the risk of Alzheimer's disease in late onset families," *Science* 261, no. 5123 (August 13, 1993): 921–23, https://doi.org/10.1126/science.8346443, PMID 8346443; W. J. Strittmatter et al., "Apolipoprotein E: high avidity binding to beta-amyloid and increased frequency of type 4 allele in late-onset familial Alzheimer disease," *Proceedings of the National Academy of Sciences of the United States of America* 90, no. 5 (March 1, 1993): 1977–81, https://doi.org/10.1073/pnas.90.5.1977, PMC 46003, PMID 8446617; I. J. Deary et al., "Cognitive change and the APOE epsilon 4 allele," *Nature* 418, no. 6901 (2002): 932, PMID 12198535.

11. D. Head et al., "Exercise engagement as a moderator of the effects of APOE genotype on amyloid deposition," *Archives of Neurology* 69 (2012): 636–43.

12. K. Talbot, "Brain insulin resistance in Alzheimer disease and its potential treatment with a mediterranean diet and GLP-1 analogues," *Psychiatric Times* (August 20, 2013): 18–21.

13. P. Crane et al., "Glucose levels and risk of dementia," *New England Journal of Medicine* 369 (August 8, 2013): 540–48.

14. Talbot, "Brain insulin resistance in Alzheimer disease."

15. G. Cooper, *The Cell: A Molecular Approach*, 2nd ed. (Sunderland, MA: Sinauer Associates, 2000), viewed online at https://www.ncbi.nlm.nih.gov/books/NBK9932/.

16. J. Busciglio et al., "Beta-amyloid fibrils induce tau phosphorylation and loss of microtubule binding," *Neuron* 14, no. 4 (April 1995): 879–88.

17. C. S. Atwood et al., "Amyloid-β: a chameleon walking in two worlds: a review of the trophic and toxic properties of amyloid-β," *Brain Research Reviews* 43, no. 1 (September 2003): 1–16.

18. Busciglio et al., "Beta-amyloid fibrils induce tau phosphorylation."

19. S. Balwinder et al., "Association of Mediterranean diet with mild cognitive impairment and Alzheimer's disease: a systematic review and meta-analysis," *Journal of Alzheimer's Disease* 39, no. 2 (2014): 271–82. See also N. Scarmeas et al., "Mediterranean diet and mild cognitive impairment," *Archives of Neurology* 66, no. 2 (2009): 216–25, https://doi.org/10.1001/archneurol.2008.536; C. Féart, C. Samieri, and P. Barberger-Gateau, "Mediterranean diet and cognitive function in older adults," *Current Opinion in Clinical Nutrition & Metabolic Care* 13, no. 1 (January 2010): 14–18, https://www.ncbi.nlm.nih.gov/pmc/articles/PMC2997798.

20. T. Manini et al., "Physical activity and maintaining physical function in older adults," *British Journal of Sports Medicine* 43 (2009): 28–31.

21. J. Holt-Lunstad et al., "Understanding the connection between spiritual well-being and physical health: an examination of ambulatory blood pressure, inflammation, blood lipids and fasting glucose," *Journal of Behavioral Medicine*

34, no. 6 (December 2011): 477–88; B. Elliott, *Forgiveness Interventions to Promote Physical Health, Forgiveness and Health: Scientific Evidence and Theories Relating Forgiveness to Better Health* (Netherlands: Springer, 2015), 271–85, accessed at http://link.springer.com/chapter/10.1007/978-94-017-9993-5_18.

22. S. Post, *Altruism and Health Perspectives from Empirical Research* (New York: Oxford University Press, 2007), 22, 26.

23. F. Zimmerman and D. Christakis, "Associations between content types of early media exposure and subsequent attentional problems," *Pediatrics* 120, no. 5 (November 5, 2007): 986–92.

24. A. Ai et al., "Research: the effect of religious-spiritual coping on positive attitudes of adult Muslim refugees from Kosovo and Bosnia," *International Journal for the Psychology of Religion* 13, no. 1 (2003): 29–47.

25. C. Féart et al., "Adherence to a Mediterranean diet, cognitive decline, and risk of dementia," *Journal of the American Medical Association* 302, no. 6 (August 2009): 638–48, https://doi.org/10.1001/jama.2009.1146. See also L. Ilanna et al., "Mediterranean diet, cognitive function, and dementia: a systematic review," *Epidemiology* 24, no. 4 (July 2013): 479–89; E. Matinez-Lapiscina et al., "Mediterranean diet improves cognition: the PREDIMED-NAVARRA randomised trial," *Journal of Neurology, Neurosurgery & Psychiatry* 84, no. 12 (December 2013): 1318–25, https://doi.org/10.1136/jnnp-2012-304792.

26. N. Barnard et al., "Dietary and lifestyle guidelines for the prevention of Alzheimer's disease," *Neurobiology of Aging* 35, no. 2 (September 2014): S74–S78.

Chapter 15 Vitamins and Supplements That Prevent Dementia

1. P. C. Beterand, J. R. O'Kusky, and S. M. Innis, "Maternal dietary (n-3) fatty acid deficiency alters neurogenesis in embryonic rat brains," *Journal of Nutrition* 136 (2006): 1570–75; E. E. Birch et al., "A randomized controlled trial of early dietary supply of long chain polyunsaturated fatty acids and mental development in term infants," *Developmental Medicine & Child Neurology* 42, no. 3 (March 2000): 174–81.

2. P. Montgomery et al., "Correction: low blood long chain omega-3 fatty acids in UK children are associated with poor cognitive performance and behavior: a cross-sectional analysis from the DOLAB study," *PLOS ONE* 8, no. 9 (2013), https://doi.org/10.1371/annotation/26c6b13f-b83a-4a3f-978a-c09d8ccf1ae2.

3. S. R. De Vriese et al., "Lowered serum n-3 polyunsaturated fatty acid (PUFA) levels predict the occurrence of postpartum depression: further evidence that lowered n-PUFAs are related to major depression," *Life Sciences* 73, no. 25 (November 7, 2003): 3181–87.

4. M. Fotuhi et al., "Fish consumption, long-chain omega-3 fatty acids and risk of cognitive decline or Alzheimer's disease: a complex association," *National Clinical Practice Neurology* 5 (2009): 140–52.

5. P. Barberger-Gateau et al., "Dietary patterns and risk of dementia: the Three City cohort study," *Neurology* 69 (2007): 1921–30.

6. E. J. Schaefer et al., "Plasma phosphatidylcholine docosahexaenoic acid content and risk of dementia and Alzheimer disease: the Framingham Heart Study," *Archives of Neurology* 63 (2006): 1545–50.

7. G. Mazereeuw et al., "Effects of omega-3 fatty acids on cognitive performance: a meta-analysis," *Neurobiology of Aging* 33 (2012): 1482.

8. Cyrus A. Raji et al., "Regular fish consumption and age-related brain gray matter loss," *American Journal of Preventive Medicine* 47, no. 4 (2014): 444–51.

9. Martha Clare Morris et al., "Association of seafood consumption, brain mercury level, and *APOE ε4* status with brain neuropathology in older adults," *Journal of the American Medical Association* 315, no. 5 (2016): 489–97, https://doi.org/10.1001/jama.2015.19451.

10. Scott Doughman et al., "Omega-3 fatty acids for nutrition and medicine: considering microalgae oil as a vegetarian source of EPA and DHA," *Current Diabetes Reviews* 3 (2007): 198–203.

11. R. J. Deckelbaum, T. S. Worgall, and T. Seo, "N-3 fatty acids and gene expression," *American Journal of Clinical Nutrition* 83, no. 6, supp. (June 2006): 1520S–25S.

12. A. Mishra, A. Chaudhary, and S. Sethi, "Oxidized n-3 fatty acids inhibit NFkappaB activation via a PPARalpha-dependent pathway," *Arteriosclerosis, Thrombosis, & Vascular Biology* 24 (2004): 1621–27. See also B. A. Narayanan et al., "Modulation of inducible nitric oxide synthase and related proinflammatory genes by the n-3 fatty acid docosahexaenoic acid in human colon cancer cells," *Cancer Research* 63 (2003): 972–79; T. Sundrarjun et al., "Effects of n-3 fatty acids on serum interleukin-6, tumour necrosis factor-alpha and soluble tumour necrosis factor receptor p55 in active rheumatoid arthritis," *Journal of International Medical Research* 32 (2004): 443–54; D. Bagga et al., "Differential effects of prostaglandin derived from n-6 and n-3 polyunsaturated fatty acids on COX-2 expression and IL-6 secretion," *Proceedings of the National Academy of Sciences of the United States of America* 100 (2003): 1751–56; T. A. Mori et al., "Effect of eicosapentaenoic acid and docosahexaenoic acid on oxidative stress and inflammatory markers in treated-hypertensive type 2 diabetic subjects," *Free Radical Biology & Medicine* 35 (2003): 772–81.

13. K. M. Nash et al., "Current perspectives on the beneficial role of ginkgo biloba in neurological and cerebrovascular disorders," *Journal of Integrative Medicine Insights* 10 (2015): 1–9.

14. J. A. Mix et al., "A double-blind, placebo-controlled, randomized trial of ginkgo biloba extract EGb 761 in a sample of cognitively intact older adults: neuropsychological findings," *Human Psychopharmacology Clinical & Experimental* 17 (2002): 267–77; R. Kaschel, "Specific memory effects of ginkgo biloba extract EGb 761 in middle-aged health volunteers," *Phytomedicine* 18 (2011): 1202–7.

15. S. T. DeKosky et al., "Ginkgo biloba for prevention of dementia: a randomized controlled trial," *Journal of the American Medical Association* 300 (2008): 2253–62.

16. B. E. Snitz et al., "Ginkgo biloba for preventing cognitive decline in older adults: a randomized trial," *Journal of the American Medical Association* 302 (2009): 2663–70.

17. H. Amieva et al., "Ginkgo biloba extract and long-term cognitive decline: a 20-year follow-up population based study," *PLOS ONE* 8 (2013): e52755.

18. S. Kohler et al., "Influence of 7-day treatment with ginkgo biloba special extract EGb 761 on bleeding time and coagulation: a randomized, placebo-controlled,

double-blind study in healthy volunteers," *Blood Coagulation & Fibrinolysis* 15 (2004): 303–9; C. D. Gardner et al., "Effects of ginkgo biloba (EGb 761) and aspirin on platelet aggregation and platelet function analysis among older adults at risk of cardiovascular disease: a randomized clinical trial," *Blood Coagulation & Fibrinolysis* 18 (2007): 787–93.

19. K. Michaelsson et al., "Plasma vitamin D and mortality in older men: a community-based prospective cohort study," *American Journal of Clinical Nutrition* 92 (2010): 841–48.

20. K. M. Saunders et al., "Annual high-dose oral vitamin D and falls and fractures in older women," *Journal of the American Medical Association* 303 (2010): 1815–22.

21. D. Durup et al., "A reverse J-shaped association of all-cause mortality with serum 25-hydroxyvitamin D in general practice, the CopD study," *Journal of Clinical Endocrinology & Metabolism* 978 (2012): 2644–52.

22. Thomas Littlejohns et al., "Vitamin D and the risk of dementia and Alzheimer disease," *Neurology* 83 (2014): 1–9.

23. E. Toffanello et al., "Vitamin D deficiency predicts cognitive decline in older men and women," *Neurology* 83, no. 24 (December 9, 2014): 2292–98.

24. A. Masoumi et al., "1 alpha, 25-dihydroxyvitamin D3 interacts with curcuminoids to stimulate amyloid-beta clearance by macrophages of Alzheimer's disease patients," *Journal of Alzheimer's Disease* 17, no. 3 (2009): 703–17.

25. K. Ono et al., "Curcumin has potent anti-amyloidogenic effects for Alzheimer's beta-amyloid fibrils in vitro," *Journal of Neuroscience Research* 75, no. 6 (March 2004): 742–50.

26. T. Hamaguchi et al., "Review: curcumin and Alzheimer's disease," *CNS Neuroscience and Therapeutics* 16, no. 5 (October 2010): 285–97.

27. J. M. Ringman et al., "A potential role of the curry spice curcumin in Alzheimer's disease," *Current Alzheimer Research* 2 (2005): 131–36; Ono et al., "Curcumin has potent anti-amyloidogenic effects."

28. M. Ganguli et al., "Apolipoprotein E polymorphism and Alzheimer disease: the Indo-US Cross-National Dementia Study," *Archives of Neurology* 57 (2000): 824–30.

29. L. Baum and A. Ng, "Curcumin interaction with copper and iron suggests one possible mechanism of action in Alzheimer's disease animal models," *Journal of Alzheimer's Disease* 6 (2004): 367–77.

30. B. L. Zhao et al., "Scavenging effect of extracts of green tea and natural antioxidants on active oxygen radicals," *Cell Biophysics* 14 (1989): 175–85; Q. Y. Wei et al., "Inhibition of lipid peroxidation and protein oxidation in rat liver mitochondria by curcumin and its analogues," *Biochimica et Biophysica Acta* 1760 (2006): 70–77.

31. J. Kim et al., "Naturally occurring phytochemicals for the prevention of Alzheimer's disease," *Journal of Neurochemistry* 112, no. 6 (March 2010): 1415–30.

32. R. A. DiSilvestro et al., "Diverse effects of a low dose supplement of lapidated curcumin in healthy middle aged people," *Nutrition Journal* 11, no. 79 (September 2012), http://nutritionj.biomedcentral.com/articles/10.1186/1475-2891-11-79.

33. S. Prasad et al., "Recent developments in delivery, bioavailability, absorption and metabolism of curcumin: the golden pigment from golden spice," *Cancer*

Research and Treatment: Official Journal of Korean Cancer Association 46, no. 1 (2014): 2–18.

34. L. Arab and A. Ang, "A cross sectional study of the association between walnut consumption and cognitive function among adult U.S. populations represented in NHANES," *Journal of Nutrition, Health and Aging* 19, no. 3 (March 2015), 284–90.

35. N. Chauhan et al., "Walnut extract inhibits the fibrillization of amyloid beta-protein, and also defibrillizes its preformed fibrils," *Current Alzheimer Research* 1, no. 3 (August 2004): 183–88.

36. S. K. Park et al., "A combination of green tea extract and l-theanine improves memory and attention in subjects with mild cognitive impairment: a double-blind placebo-controlled study," *Journal of Medicinal Food* 14 (2011): 334–43.

37. K. Rezai-Zadeh et al., "Green tea epigallocatechin-3-gallate (EGCG) reduces beta-amyloid mediated cognitive impairment and modulates tau pathology in Alzheimer transgenic mice," *Brain Research* 1214 (2008): 177–87; R. J. Williams and J. P. Spencer, "Flavonoids, cognition, and dementia: actions, mechanisms, and potential therapeutic utility for Alzheimer disease," *Free Radical Biology & Medicine* 52 (2012): 35–45.

38. S. Kuriyama et al., "Green tea consumption and cognitive function: a cross-sectional study from the Tsurugaya Project 1," *American Journal of Clinical Nutrition* 83 (2006): 355–61; T. P. Ng et al., "Tea consumption and cognitive impairment and decline in older Chinese adults," *American Journal of Clinical Nutrition* 88 (2008): 224–31.

39. L. Feng et al., "Cognitive function and tea consumption in community dwelling older Chinese in Singapore," *Journal of Nutrition, Health and Aging* 14 (2010): 433–38.

40. S. Borgwardt et al., "Neural effects of green tea extract on dorsolateral prefrontal cortex," *European Journal of Clinical Nutrition* 66 (2012): 1187–92.

41. A. M. Owen et al., "N-back working memory paradigm: a meta-analysis of normative functional neuroimaging studies," *Human Brain Mapping* 25 (2005): 46–59. See also C. Rottschy et al., "Modelling neural correlates of working memory: a coordinate-based meta-analysis," *Neuroimage* 60 (2012): 830–46; L. Deserno et al., "Reduced prefrontal-parietal effective connectivity and working memory deficits in schizophrenia," *Journal of Neuroscience* 32 (2012): 12–20; A. Schmidt et al., "Green tea extract enhances parieto-frontal connectivity during working memory processing," *Psychopharmacology* 31, no. 19 (October 2014): 3879–88.

42. Schmidt et al., "Green tea extract enhances parieto-frontal connectivity."

43. R. Hartman et al., "Pomegranate juice decreases amyloid load and improves behavior in a mouse model of Alzheimer's disease," *Neurobiology of Disease* 24, no. 3 (December 2006): 506–15.

44. Q. Dai et al., "Fruit and vegetable juices and Alzheimer's disease: the Kame Project," *American Journal of Medicine* 119, no. 9 (September 2006): 751–59.

45. C. Gau et al., "Pomegranate juice is potentially better than apple juice in improving antioxidant function in elderly subjects," *Nutrition Research* 28, no. 2 (February 2008): 72–77.

46. L. Rojanathammanne et al., "Pomegranate polyphenols and extract inhibit nuclear factor of activated T-cell activity and microglial activation in vitro and

in a transgenic mouse model of Alzheimer disease," *Journal of Nutrition* 143, no. 5 (May 1, 2013): 597–605.

47. N. Freedman et al., "Association of coffee drinking with total and cause-specific mortality," *New England Journal of Medicine* 366 (May 17, 2012): 1891–1904, https://doi.org/10.1056/NEJMoa1112010.

48. A. Cano-Marquina et al., "The impact of coffee on health," *Maturitus, the European Menopause Journal* 75, no. 1 (May 2013): 7–21.

49. J. N. Wu et al., "Coffee consumption and risk of coronary heart diseases: a meta-analysis of 21 prospective cohort studies," *International Journal of Cardiology* 137 (2009): 216–25. See also F. Natella et al., "Coffee drinking induces incorporation of phenolic acids into LDL and increases the resistance of LDL to ex vivo oxidation in humans," *American Journal of Clinical Nutrition* 86 (2007): 604–9; J. A. Gómez-Ruiz, D. S. Leake, and J. M. Ames, "In vitro antioxidant activity of coffee compounds and their metabolites," *Journal of Agricultural & Food Chemistry* 55 (2007): 6962–69; M. Nardini et al., "Inhibition of human low-density lipoprotein oxidation by caffeic acid and other hydroxycinnamic acid derivatives," *Free Radical Biology & Medicine* 19 (1995): 541–52; M. Montagnana, E. J. Favaloro, and G. Lippi, "Coffee intake and cardiovascular disease: virtue does not take center stage," *Seminars in Thrombosis & Hemostasis* 38 (2012): 164–77.

50. Wu et al., "Coffee consumption and risk of coronary heart diseases."

51. E. Mostofsky et al., "Habitual coffee consumption and risk of heart failure: a dose–response meta-analysis," *Circulation: Heart Failure* 5 (July 2012): 401–5, https://doi.org/10.1161/CIRCHEARTFAILURE.112.967299.

52. S. C. Larsson and N. Orsini, "Coffee consumption and risk of stroke: a dose-response meta-analysis of prospective studies," *American Journal of Epidemiology* 174 (2011): 993–1001.

53. S. C. Larsson, J. Virtamo, and A. Wolk, "Coffee consumption and risk of stroke in women," *Stroke* 42 (2011): 908–12.

54. R. Huxley et al., "Coffee, decaffeinated coffee, and tea consumption in relation to incident type 2 diabetes mellitus: a systematic review with meta-analysis," *Archives of Internal Medicine* 169 (2009): 2053–63; D. S. Sartorelli et al., "Differential effects of coffee on the risk of type 2 diabetes according to meal consumption in a French cohort of women: the E3N/EPIC cohort study," *American Journal of Clinical Nutrition* 91 (2010): 1002–112.

55. B. Cheng et al., "Coffee components inhibit amyloid formation of human islet amyloid polypeptide in vitro: possible link between coffee consumption and diabetes mellitus," *Journal of Agricultural & Food Chemistry* 59, no. 24 (2011): 13147–55.

56. Y. Je et al., "A prospective cohort study of coffee consumption and risk of endometrial cancer over a 26-year follow-up," *Cancer, Epidemiology, Biomarkers & Prevention* 20 (2011): 1–9.

57. K. M. Wilson et al., "Coffee consumption and prostate cancer risk and progression in the Health Professionals Follow-Up Study," *Journal of the National Cancer Institute* 8, no. 103 (2011): 876–84.

58. F. Turati et al., "Coffee and cancers of the upper digestive and respiratory tracts: meta-analyses of observational studies," *Annals of Oncology* 22 (2011): 536–44; C. Galeone et al., "Coffee and tea intake and risk of head and neck

cancer: pooled analysis in the international head and neck cancer epidemiology consortium," *Cancer Epidemiology, Biomarkers, & Prevention* 19 (2010): 1723–36.

59. F. Song, A. A. Qureshi, and J. Han, "Increased caffeine intake is associated with reduced risk of basal cell carcinoma of the skin," *Cancer Research* 72 (2012): 3282–89.

60. J. Li et al., "Coffee consumption modifies risk of estrogen-receptor negative breast cancer," *Breast Cancer Research* 13 (2011): R49.

61. Je et al., "A prospective cohort study of coffee consumption and risk of endometrial cancer"; Turati et al., "Coffee and cancers of the upper digestive and respiratory tracts."

62. M. Eskelinene et al., "Caffeine as a protective factor in dementia and Alzheimer's disease," *Journal of Alzheimer's Disease* 20, no. S1 (2010): 167–74.

63. C. Cao et al., "High blood caffeine levels in MCI linked to lack of progression to dementia," *Journal of Alzheimer's Disease* 30 (2012): 559–72.

64. G. Arendash et al., "Caffeine and coffee as therapeutics against Alzheimer's disease," *Journal of Alzheimer's Disease* 20, no. S1 (2010): 117–26.

65. C. Chuanhai et al., "Caffeine synergizes with another coffee component to increase plasma GCSF: linkage to cognitive benefits in Alzheimer's mice," *Journal of Alzheimer's Disease* 25, no. 2 (2011): 323–35.

66. X. Guo et al., "Sweetened beverages, coffee, and tea and depression risk among older US adults," *PLOS ONE* 9, no. 4 (2014): e94715, https://doi.org/10.1371/journal.pone.0094715.

67. A. Miller, V. Maletic, and C. Raison, "Inflammation and its discontents: the role of cytokines in the pathophysiology of major depression," *Biological Psychiatry* 65, no. 9 (May 1, 2009): 732–41.

68. J. S. Saczynski et al., "Depressive symptoms and risk of dementia," *Neurology* 75, no. 1 (July 6, 2010): 35–41.

69. T. Hamza et al., "Genome-wide gene-environment study identifies glutamate receptor gene *GRIN2A* as a Parkinson's disease modifier gene via interaction with coffee," *PlOS Genetics* (August 18, 2011), http://journals.plos.org/plosgenetics/article?id=10.1371/journal.pgen.1002237.

70. K. Kaufman et al., "Caffeinated beverages and decreased seizure control," *Seizure* 12, no. 7 (October 2003): 519–21.

71. P. E. Hinkle et al., "Use of caffeine to lengthen seizures in ECT," *American Journal of Psychiatry* 144, no. 9 (September 1987): 1143–48; "Caffeine Augmentation of ECT," *American Journal of Psychiatry* 147, no. 5 (May 1990): 579–85.

72. M. Wilson, "Caffeine induced changes in cerebral circulation," *Stroke* 16 (1985): 814–17; E. Casiglia et al., "Haemodynamic effects of coffee and caffeine in normal volunteers: a placebo-controlled clinical study," *Journal of Internal Medicine* 229, no. 6 (June 1991): 501–4; K. Lotfi et al., "The effect of caffeine on the human macular circulation," *Investigative Ophthalmology & Visual Science* 32 (November 1991): 3028–32; J. Daniels et al., "Effects of caffeine on blood pressure, heart rate, and forearm blood flow during dynamic leg exercise," *Journal of Applied Physiology* 85, no. 1 (July 1, 1998): 154–59.

73. C. L. Hawco et al., "A Maple Syrup Extract Prevents β-Amyloid Aggregation," *Canadian Journal of Neurological Sciences* 43, no. 1 (2016): 198–201.

74. M. Meydani, "Vitamin E," *Lancet* 345 (1995): 170–75; J. M. Upston, A. C. Terentis, and R. Stocker, "Tocopherol-mediated peroxidation of lipoproteins:

implications for vitamin E as a potential antiatherogenic supplement," *FASEB Journal* 13 (1999): 977–94.

75. K. F. Gey et al., "Inverse correlation between plasma vitamin E and mortality from ischemic heart disease in cross-cultural epidemiology," *American Journal of Clinical Nutrition* 53, no. 1, supp. (January 1991): 326S–34S.

76. M. J. Stampfer et al., "Vitamin E consumption and the risk of coronary disease in women," *New England Journal of Medicine* 328 (1993): 1444–49; E. B. Rimm et al., "Vitamin E consumption and the risk of coronary heart disease in men," *New England Journal of Medicine* 328 (1993): 1450–56.

77. R. E. Patterson et al., "Vitamin supplements and cancer risk: the epidemiologic evidence," *Cancer Causes Control* 8 (1997): 786–802.

78. M. Lee et al., "Vitamin E in the primary prevention of cardiovascular disease and cancer: the Women's Health Study: a randomized controlled trial," *Journal of the American Medical Association* 294, no. 1 (2005): 56–65.

79. E. Miller et al., "Meta-analysis: high-dosage vitamin E supplementation may increase all-cause mortality," *Annals of Internal Medicine* 142, no. 1 (2005): 37–46.

80. Rimm et al., "Vitamin E consumption and the risk of coronary heart disease in men."

81. S. Lippman et al., "Effect of selenium and vitamin E on risk of prostate cancer and other cancers: the Selenium and Vitamin E Cancer Prevention Trial (SELECT)," *Journal of the American Medical Association* 301, no. 1 (2009): 39–51.

82. S. Sung et al., "Early vitamin E supplementation in young but not aged mice reduces AB levels and amyloid deposition in a transgenic model of Alzheimer's disease," *FASEB Journal* 18, no. 2 (February 2004): 323–25.

83. M. J. Engelhart et al., "Dietary intake of antioxidants and risk of Alzheimer disease," *Journal of the American Medical Association* 287 (2002): 3223–29; M. C. Morris et al., "Dietary intake of antioxidant nutrients and the risk of incident Alzheimer's disease in a biracial community study," *Journal of the American Medical Association* 287 (2002): 3230–37.

84. M. G. Isaac, R. Quinn, and N. Tabet, "Vitamin E for Alzheimer's disease and mild cognitive impairment," *Cochrane Database of Systematic Reviews*, no. 3 (July 16, 2008), art. no.: CD002854, https://doi.org/10.1002/14651858.CD002854.pub2; Shelly Gray et al., "Antioxidant vitamin supplement use and risk of dementia or Alzheimer's disease in older adults," *Journal of American Geriatric Society* 56, no. 2 (February 2008): 291–95.

85. F. Harrison et al., "Vitamin C function in the brain: vital role of the ascorbate transporter SVCT2," *Free Radical Biology and Medicine* 46, no. 6 (March 15, 2009): 719–30.

86. M. Morris, "Diet and Alzheimer's disease: what the evidence shows," *Medscape General Medicine* 6, no. 1 (2004): 48.

87. D. Berk et al., "N-acetylcysteine in psychiatry: current therapeutic evidence and potential mechanisms of action," *Journal of Psychiatry & Neuroscience* 36, no. 2 (March 2011): 78–86.

88. P. Moreira et al., "Lipoic acid and N-acetyl cysteine decrease mitochondrial-related oxidative stress in Alzheimer disease patient fibroblasts," *Journal of Alzheimer's Disease* 12, no. 2 (2007): 195–206.

89. M. Banaclocha, "Therapeutic potential of N-acetylcysteine in age-related mitochondrial neurodegenerative diseases," *Medical Hypotheses* 56, no. 4 (April 2001): 472–77.

90. M. Martinez et al., "N-acetylcysteine delays age-associated memory impairment in mice: role in synaptic mitochondria," *Brain Research* 855, no. 1 (February 7, 2000): 100–106.

91. R. Oh and D. L. Brown, "Vitamin B12 deficiency," *American Family Physician* 67, no. 5 (2003): 979–86.

92. H. Tiemeier et al., "Vitamin B12, folate, and homocysteine in depression: the Rotterdam Study," *American Journal of Psychiatry* 159, no. 12 (December 2002): 2099–101; S. Lewis et al., "The thermolabile variant of MTHFR is associated with depression in the British Women's Heart and Health Study and a meta-analysis," *Molecular Psychiatry* 11 (2006): 352–60.

93. P. Kirke et al., "Maternal plasma folate and vitamin B12 are independent risk factors for neural tube defects," *QJM: An International Journal of Medicine* 86, no. 11 (November 1993): 703–8.

94. P. Stover, "Physiology of folate and vitamin B12 in health and disease," *Nutrition Reviews* 62, no. 6, pt. 2 (June 2004): S3–12.

95. M. Cravo et al., "Hyperhomocysteinemia in chronic alcoholism: correlation with folate, vitamin B-12, and vitamin B-6 status," *American Journal of Clinical Nutrition* 63, no. 2 (February 1996): 220–24.

96. H. Wang et al., "Vitamin B_{12} and folate in relation to the development of Alzheimer's disease," *Neurology* 56, no. 9 (May 8, 2001): 1188–94; I. Kruman et al., "Folic acid deficiency and homocysteine impair DNA repair in hippocampal neurons and sensitize them to amyloid toxicity in experimental models of Alzheimer's disease," *Journal of Neuroscience* 22, no. 5 (March 1, 2002): 1752–62.

97. Stover, "Physiology of folate and vitamin B12 in health and disease."

98. Alan L. Miller, "The methylation, neurotransmitter, and antioxidant connections between folate and depression," *Alternative Medicine Review* 13, no. 3 (September 2008): 216–26.

99. R. Clarke et al., "Folate, vitamin B12, and serum total homocysteine levels in confirmed Alzheimer disease," *Archives of Neurology* 55, no. 11 (1998): 1449–55. See also P. Quadri et al., "Homocysteine, folate, and vitamin B-12 in mild cognitive impairment, Alzheimer disease, and vascular dementia," *American Journal of Clinical Nutrition* 80, no. 1 (July 2004): 114–22; M. Haan et al., "Homocysteine, B vitamins, and the incidence of dementia and cognitive impairment: results from the Sacramento Area Latino Study on Aging," *American Journal of Clinical Nutrition* 85, no. 2 (February 2007): 511–17; M. Ramos, "Low folate status is associated with impaired cognitive function and dementia in the Sacramento Area Latino Study on Aging," *American Journal of Clinincal Nutrition* 82, no. 6 (December 2005): 1346–52.

100. A. Vogiatzoglou et al., "Vitamin B12 status and rate of brain volume loss in community-dwelling elderly," *Neurology* 71, no. 11 (September 9, 2008): 826–32.

101. E. Andres et al., "Vitamin B_{12} (cobalamin) deficiency in elderly patients," *Canadian Medical Association Journal* 171, no. 3 (August 3, 2004), https://doi.org/10.1503/cmaj.1031155.

102. C. Hong et al., "Anemia and risk of dementia in older adults," *Neurology* 81, no. 6 (August 6, 2013): 528–33; M. Andro et al., "Anaemia and cognitive performances in the elderly: a systematic review," *European Journal of Neurology* 20, no. 9 (September 2013): 1234–40.

103. S. P. Marcuard, L. Albernaz, and P. G. Khazanie, "Omeprazole therapy causes malabsorption of cyanocobalamin (vitamin B12)," *Annals of Internal Medicine* 120 (1994): 211–15; J. R. Saltzman et al., "Effect of hypochlorhydria due to omeprazole treatment or atrophic gastritis on protein-bound vitamin B12 absorption," *Journal of the American College of Nutrition* 13 (1994): 584–91.

104. W. P. den Elzen et al., "Long-term use of proton pump inhibitors and vitamin B12 status in elderly individuals," *Alimentary Pharmacology & Therapeutics* 27, no. 6 (2008): 491–97. See also C. W. Howden, "Vitamin B12 levels during prolonged treatment with proton pump inhibitors," *Journal of Clinical Gastroenterology* 30 (2000): 29–33; P. N. Maton et al., "Long-term efficacy and safety of omeprazole in patients with Zollinger-Ellison syndrome: a prospective study," *Gastroenterology* 97 (1989): 827–36.

105. B. Termanini et al., "Effect of long-term gastric acid suppressive therapy on serum vitamin B12 levels in patients with Zollinger-Ellison syndrome," *American Journal of Medicine* 104 (1998): 422–30.

106. B. E. Schenk et al., "Atrophic gastritis during long-term omeprazole therapy affects serum vitamin B12 levels," *Alimentary Pharmacology & Therapeutics* 13 (1999): 1343–46.

107. M. Tsai et al., "Polygenic influence on plasma homocysteine: association of two prevalent mutations, the 844ins68 of cystathionine β-synthase and $A_{2756}G$ of methionine synthase, with lowered plasma homocysteine levels," *Atherosclerosis* 149, no. 1 (March 2000): 131–37.

108. Tsai et al., "Polygenic influence on plasma homocysteine." See also D. Mischoulon et al., "Prevalence of MTHFR C677T and MS A2756G polymorphisms in major depressive disorder, and their impact on response to fluoxetine treatment," *CNS Spectrums* 17, no. 2 (June 2012): 76–86; S. Lewis et al., "The thermolabile variant of MTHFR is associated with depression in the British Women's Heart and Health Study and a meta-analysis," *Molecular Psychiatry* 11 (2006): 352–60.

109. U. Das, "Folic acid and polyunsaturated fatty acids improve cognitive function and prevent depression, dementia, and Alzheimer's disease—But how and why?," *Prostaglandins, Leukotrienes and Essential Fatty Acids* 78, no. 1 (January 2008): 11–19.

110. D. van Diermen et al., "Monoamine oxidase inhibition by Rhodiola rosea L. roots," *Journal of Ethnopharmacology* 122, no. 2 (March 18, 2009): 397–401.

111. Seyed Fazel Nabavi et al., "*Rhodiola rosea* L. and Alzheimer's disease: from farm to pharmacy," *Phytotherapy Research* 30, no. 4 (April 2016): 532–39, https://doi.org/10.1002/ptr.5569; M. Ganzera, Y. Yayla, and I. A. Khan, "Analysis of the marker compounds of *Rhodiola rosea* L. (golden root) by reversed phase high performance liquid chromatography," *Chemical & Pharmaceutical Bulletin* 49 (2001): 465–67.

112. D. R. Palumbo et al., "*Rhodiola rosea* extract protects human cortical neurons against glutamate and hydrogen peroxide-induced cell death through reduction in the accumulation of intracellular calcium," *Phytotherapy Research*

26, no. 6 (June 2012): 878–83. See also Ze-Qiang Qu et al., "Pretreatment with *Rhodiola rosea* extract reduces cognitive impairment induced by intracerebroventricular streptozotocin in rats: implication of anti-oxidative and neuroprotective effects," *Biomedical and Environmental Sciences* 22, no. 4 (August 2009): 318–26; Y. Lee et al., "Anti-inflammatory and neuroprotective effects of constituents isolated from *Rhodiola rosea*," *Evidence-Based Complementary and Alternative Medicine* 2013 (2013), http://dx.doi.org/10.1155/2013/514049.

113. E. M. Olsson et al., "A randomised, double-blind, placebo-controlled, parallel-group study of the standardised extract SHR-5 of the roots of *Rhodiola rosea* in the treatment of subjects with stress-related fatigue," *Planta Medica* 75, no. 2 (2009): 105–12, https://doi.org/10.1055/s-0028-1088346.

114. D. V. Gospodaryov et al., "Lifespan extension and delay of age-related functional decline caused by *Rhodiola rosea* depends on dietary macronutrient balance," *Longevity & Healthspan* 2, no. 5 (2013), https://doi.org/10.1186/2046 -2395-2-5. See also G. Mao et al., "Salidroside protects human fibroblast cells from premature senescence induced by H_2O_2 partly through modulating oxidative status," *Mechanisms of Ageing and Development* 131, nos. 11–12 (November–December 2010): 723–31; G. Mao et al., "Protective role of salidroside against aging in a mouse model induced by D-galactose," *Biomedical and Environmental Sciences* 23, no. 2 (April 2010): 161–66.

115. G. Aslanyan et al., "Double-blind, placebo-controlled, randomised study of single dose effects of ADAPT-232 on cognitive functions," *Phytomedicine* 17, no. 7 (June 2010): 494–99.

116. D. van Diermen et al., "Monoamine oxidase inhibition by Rhodiola rosea L. roots," *Journal of Ethnopharmacology* 122, no. 2 (March 18, 2009): 397–401; B. Hillhouse et al., "Acetylcholine esterase inhibitors in *Rhodiola rosea*," *Pharmaceutical Biology* 42, no. 1 (2004): 68–72.

117. B. Imtiaz et al., "Postmenopausal hormone therapy and Alzheimer disease: a prospective cohort study," *Neurology* 88, no. 11 (March 14, 2017): 1062–68.

118. H. Shao et al., "Hormone therapy and Alzheimer disease dementia: new findings from the Cache County Study," *Neurology* 79, no. 18 (October 30, 2012): 1846–52.

119. J. E. Manson et al., "Menopausal hormone therapy and health outcomes during the intervention and extended poststopping phases of the Women's Health Initiative randomized trials," *Journal of the American Medical Association* 310 (2013): 1353–68; H. N. Hodis et al., "ELITE Research Group. Vascular effects of early versus late postmenopausal treatment with estradiol," *New England Journal of Medicine* 374 (March 31, 2016): 1221–31.

Chapter 16 Risk Factors for Dementia and How to Reduce the Risk

1. F. Forette et al., "The prevention of dementia with antihypertensive treatment: new evidence from the Systolic Hypertension in Europe (Syst-Eur) Study," *Archives of Internal Medicine* 162, no. 18 (2002): 2046–52, https://doi.org/10.1001 /archinte.162.18.2046.

2. J. S. Saczynski et al., "Depressive symptoms and risk of dementia," *Neurology* 75, no. 1 (July 6, 2010): 35–41.

Timothy R. Jennings, MD, is a board-certified Christian psychiatrist, master psychopharmacologist, international speaker, Distinguished Fellow of the American Psychiatric Association, and Fellow of the Southern Psychiatric Association. Dr. Jennings obtained his MD degree in 1990 from the University of Tennessee College of Medicine in Memphis, Tennessee. He completed psychiatric residency at D. D. Eisenhower Army Medical Center in Augusta, Georgia, and has served as the Division Psychiatrist for the 3rd Infantry Division. Dr. Jennings is president and founder of Come and Reason Ministries and has served as president of the Southern and Tennessee Psychiatric Associations. He is married and lives in Chattanooga, Tennessee, where he is in private practice.

Dr. Jennings is the author of the following books:

Could It Be This Simple? A Biblical Model for Healing the Mind
The God-Shaped Brain: How Changing Your View of God Transforms Your Life
The Journal of the Watcher
The Remedy: A New Testament Expanded Paraphrase in Everyday English
The God-Shaped Heart: How Correctly Understanding God's Love Transforms Us

Dr. Jennings's lectures and written material can be found at www.comeandreason.com.

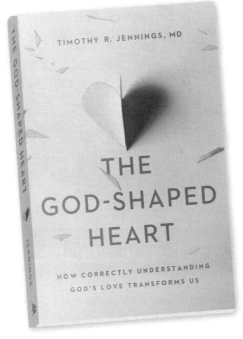

Connect with
Dr. Tim Jennings

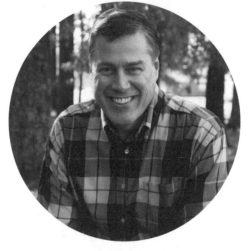

Book **Tim** for your event!

Dr. Jennings has spent more than two decades researching the interface between biblical principles and modern brain science and is a highly sought-after lecturer and international speaker. Email **Requests@ComeandReason.com** with speaking inquiries.

— Host an Aging Brain Seminar! —

Visit **AgingBrainBook.com** to learn more about Dr. Jennings's seminars.

Learn more about your health!

Dr. Jennings has many resources available (videos, podcasts, blogs, articles, and more) at **TimJenningsMD.com,** and information about his psychiatric practice can be found at **TMSChattanooga.com.**

 TimJenningsMD   ComeandReasonMinistries

 ComeandReasonMinistries   Come and Reason Ministries

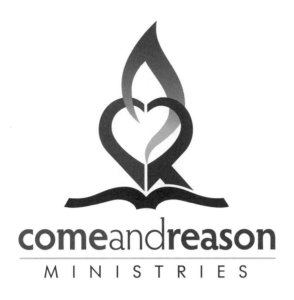

comeandreason
M I N I S T R I E S

Come and Reason Ministries was founded by Christian psychiatrist Dr. Tim Jennings. Our mission is to help you hone your mental faculties by providing materials that integrate Scripture, science, and experience to reveal the beauty of God's character of love so you can grow in your relationship with God.

Join Dr. Tim Jennings for Come and Reason Ministries' weekly Bible study as he answers tough biblical questions by applying God's design law.

Visit **ComeandReason.com** to find out how to stream live, or watch directly from the app. Search Come and Reason from your device's app store.

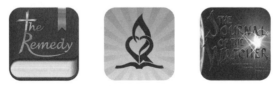

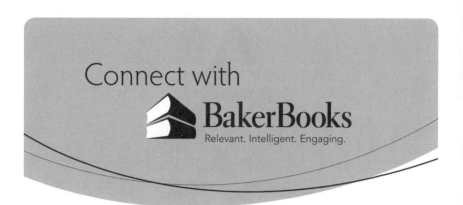

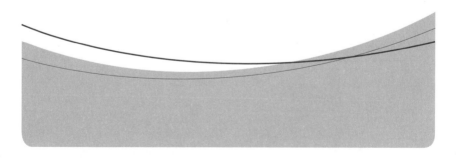